T0185588

Hair Transplant Surgery and Platelet Rich Plasma

Linda N. Lee

Editor

Hair Transplant Surgery and Platelet Rich Plasma

Evidence-Based Essentials

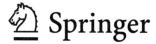 Springer

Editor
Linda N. Lee, MD, FACS
Facial Plastic and Reconstructive Surgery
Assistant Professor, Harvard Medical School
Massachusetts Eye and Ear
Associate Chief of Plastic Surgery, Harvard Vanguard Medical Associates
Boston, MA
USA

ISBN 978-3-030-54650-2   ISBN 978-3-030-54648-9   (eBook)
https://doi.org/10.1007/978-3-030-54648-9

This Springer imprint is published by the registered company Springer Nature Switzerland AG
The registered company address is: Gewerbestrasse 11, 6330 Cham, Switzerland

I dedicate this book to my incredible family: Jason, Connor, & Dylan. Thank you for your love and support that enabled this important project to be completed.

Foreword

A practically focused handbook that is rooted in evidence-based literature has been very much needed in the area of hair transplant surgery and ancillary treatments. It is also very hard to accomplish. However, that is exactly what Dr. Lee and her coauthors have done in this new textbook for beginners to advanced surgeons in this rapidly evolving field. Balancing a broad set of procedures with key details, pearls, and pitfalls, the text addresses many core practitioners' questions of "how to do it" and also answers the more important issues of why, when, and for whom. Written in an easy-to-follow style, with photographs and checklists, Dr. Lee has made both simple and intricate procedures accessible and clear.

The handbook proceeds in a logical order. It starts with a review of relevant anatomy and physiology and medical treatments for alopecia. The next part begins with a clear description of indications and contraindications for patient selection in hair transplantation and progresses to surgical basics, key components like designing the hairline, and detailed illustrations of follicular unit techniques. It covers details such as local anesthesia and postoperative instructions, ancillary techniques around the beard and eyebrow, and use of plasma-rich protein, which are critical for the surgeon but often overlooked in similar texts. There are abundant references to guide the reader to deeper investigations into technical nuances or outcomes reviews. The contributing authors include well-known experts from both academic and community-based practices.

In developing this textbook, Dr. Lee and her co-authors have found the right balance between practicality and detail. It lives up to its promise of providing the "evidence-based essentials." This textbook is highly recommended to practitioners of all levels, trainees, and clinical staff.

Richard E. Gliklich, MD
Leffenfield Professor, Harvard Medical School
Division of Facial Plastic and Reconstructive Surgery
Department of Otolaryngology-Head and Neck Surgery
Massachusetts Eye and Ear
Boston, MA, USA

Preface

Modern hair transplantation combines innovative techniques with advanced artistry to achieve natural results. The accessibility and prevalence of evidence-based outcomes data has contributed to an increase in the number of patients pursuing hair loss treatment. In recent decades, the treatment algorithm for hair loss has evolved from standard single surgical approach to multiple surgical and non-surgical options, customized to the individual. Hair loss patients and clinicians work together to create a treatment plan which may include medical therapies, minimally invasive procedures such as platelet-rich plasma (PRP), and surgical hair transplantation. Both follicular unit extraction (FUE) and follicular unit transplant (FUT) techniques offer unique advantages for each patient. Additionally, hairline-lowering surgeries remain a distinct option for patients to effectively restore a more youthful hairline.

Perhaps because patients are so highly motivated to pursue hair loss treatments, the online community is fraught with anecdotal, non-evidence-based treatments that can be costly and ineffective. This textbook is dedicated to reviewing evidence-based treatment options for hair loss to help clinicians accurately identify the optimal treatment plan for each patient. Risks of each treatment and patient selection criteria are discussed to help both clinicians and patients save time and avoid costly treatments that have not demonstrated success.

The chapters in this book have been authored by leading experts in facial plastic surgery and dermatology, each of whom specializes in hair restoration. The content has been specifically collated to concisely review essential topics to help readers understand the physiology of hair loss, the natural cycle of hair regrowth, and medical factors that guide the treatment plan optimal to each patient. Postoperative patient instructions and realistic patient expectations are discussed. Authors share important cautionary tips to avoid rare complications of hair transplant surgery. Surgical pearls are offered to help clinicians achieve the most natural-appearing results for their patients.

I extend sincere thanks to the authors for sharing an overwhelming wealth of expertise in this concise medical textbook. Through collaboration with physicians dedicated to evidence-based, safe, and successful treatment, we will continue to advance the field of hair restoration and help patients improve their quality of life. The body of literature that exists for hair restoration is steadily growing, and I am proud to be a part of this outstanding medical resource which can help train hair restoration surgeons for the future.

Boston, MA, USA   Linda N. Lee

Contents

Contributors

Anthony Bared, MD, FACS South Miami Hospital, Department of Otolaryngology, Miami, FL, USA

Prabhat K. Bhama, MD, MPH, FACS University of Hawaii John A. Burns School of Medicine, University of Washington School of Medicine, Seattle, WA, USA

Jenny X. Chen, MD Massachusetts Eye and Ear, Department of Otolaryngology-Head and Neck Surgery, Harvard Medical School, Boston, MA, USA

Michael S. Chow, MD New York University, Department of Otolaryngology – Head and Neck Surgery, New York, NY, USA

Chen Chen Costelloe, MD Brigham Healthcare, Department of Anesthesiology, Harvard Medical School, Boston, MA, USA

Lisa Ishii, MD, MHS Johns Hopkins Hospital, Department of Otolaryngology, Lutherville, MD, USA

Natalie Justicz, MD Massachusetts Eye and Ear, Department of Otolaryngology-Head and Neck Surgery, Harvard Medical School, Boston, MA, USA

Amit Kochhar, MD Facial Plastic and Reconstructive Surgery, Pacific Neuroscience Institute, Santa Monica, CA, USA

Linda N. Lee, MD, FACS Facial Plastic and Reconstructive Surgery, Assistant Professor, Harvard Medical School, Massachusetts Eye and Ear, Associate Chief of Plastic Surgery, Harvard Vanguard Medical Associates, Boston, MA, USA

Michael C. Lubrano, MD, MPH South Shore Hospital, Department of Anesthesiology & Pain Medicine, South Weymouth, MA, USA

Dustin H. Marks, BS Massachusetts General Hospital, Department of Dermatology, Harvard Medical School, Boston, MA, USA

Sarina K. Mueller, MD Friedrich-Alexander-Universität Erlangen-Nürnberg (FAU), Department of Otolaryngology, Head and Neck Surgery, Erlangen, Germany

Sahar Nadimi, MD Department of Otolaryngology-Head and Neck Surgery, Loyola University Medical Center, Maywood, IL, USA

Private Practice in Oakbrook Terrace, Maywood, IL, USA

Jean-Phillip Okhovat, MD, MPH Massachusetts General Hospital, Department of Dermatology, Harvard Medical School, Boston, MA, USA

Samuel L. Oyer, MD Facial Plastic & Reconstructive Surgery, University of Virginia, Charlottesville, VA, USA

Dylan Russell, MD General Surgery Resident, Tripler Army Medical Center, Honolulu, HI, USA

Maryanne Makredes Senna, MD MGH Hair Loss Clinic; Hair Academic Innovative Research (HAIR) Unit, Department of Dermatology, Massachusetts General Hospital, Harvard Medical School, Boston, MA, USA

Ryan M. Smith, MD Facial Plastic and Reconstructive Surgery, Rush University Medical Center, Otorhinolaryngology – Head and Neck Surgery, Chicago, IL, USA

Tymon Tai, MD Keck School of Medicine of USC, USC Caruso Department of Otolaryngology Head and Neck Surgery, Los Angeles, CA, USA

Joe K. Tung, MD, MBA Harvard Medical School, Boston, MA, USA

Matthew J. Urban, MD Facial Plastic and Reconstructive Surgery, Rush University Medical Center, Otorhinolaryngology – Head and Neck Surgery, Chicago, IL, USA

Mariko R. Yasuda, MD Massachusetts General Hospital, Department of Dermatology, Harvard Medical School, Boston, MA, USA

Robert Jason Yong, MD, MBA Division of Pain Medicine, Department of Anesthesiology and Pain Medicine, Brigham and Women's Hospital, Harvard Medical School, Boston, MA, USA

Anatomy and Physiology of the Hair Cycle

Joe K. Tung and Mariko R. Yasuda

Types of Hair

Hair may vary considerably in length, width, quantity, and distribution of follicles depending on its type and location on the human body. The two main types of hair are terminal hair and vellus hair. Terminal hairs are normally thicker and longer, with hair shaft diameters greater than 0.06 mm and hair bulbs rooted deeply in the subcutaneous tissue. On the other hand, vellus hairs are usually only 1–2 mm in length and have thinner shafts measuring less than 0.03 mm in diameter. Their bulbs are located in the upper portion of the dermis, and they are characteristically more hypopigmented than the baseline hair color. Vellus hair is typically more noticeable on women and children because men tend to have more terminal body hair [1].

Prior to puberty, terminal hair is found on the scalp, eyelashes, and eyebrows, whereas vellus hair covers the majority of the rest of the body to protect the skin and keep the body warm. During puberty, hormonal changes—particularly an increase in androgens—cause vellus hairs to enlarge and become terminal hairs in certain parts of the body. This transformation is most noticeable on the underarm and pubic areas of men and women as well as on beards in men. Androgens act by lengthening the period of time the hair is growing and by modulating the activities of hair cells, keratinocytes, and melanocytes [2].

Paradoxically, terminal hairs on the scalp can also revert to vellus-like hairs later in life under the influence of androgens, such as in individuals with androgenic alopecia. This androgen effect varies based on the hair follicle location. Typically, hair in the frontal scalp is more sensitive than hair in the occipital scalp [3]. These areas differ with respect to their metabolism of androgen, the number of androgen receptors present, and the response of cells to androgens [4]. Some cells secrete

J. K. Tung (✉)
Harvard Medical School, Boston, MA, USA

M. R. Yasuda
Massachusetts General Hospital, Department of Dermatology, Harvard Medical School, Boston, MA, USA

© Springer Nature Switzerland AG 2020
L. N. Lee (ed.), *Hair Transplant Surgery and Platelet Rich Plasma*,
https://doi.org/10.1007/978-3-030-54648-9_1

mitogens in response to androgens and consequently promote hair growth, whereas other cells secrete inhibitory factors and therefore inhibit hair growth [5].

Structure of Hair Follicles

Regardless of their location, terminal hair follicles all have a similar basic structure and can be divided into three main regions: the lower portion (hair bulb and supra-bulbar zone), the middle portion (isthmus), and the upper portion (infundibulum). The lower portion extends from the hair bulb—located in the subcutaneous fat—to the inferior insertion point of the arrector pili muscle, which functions to erect hair under sympathetic nervous system control. The middle portion extends from the insertion of the arrector pili muscle inferiorly to the entrance of the sebaceous gland duct superiorly. The isthmus serves as a significant transitional zone for follicular keratinization. The upper portion extends from the entrance of the sebaceous duct to the follicular orifice and merges with the surface epidermis. Whereas the lower portion of the hair follicle regresses and regenerates on a cyclical basis, the isthmus and infundibulum remain permanent for each follicle [1].

The hair follicle, arrector pili muscle, and sebaceous gland together compose the pilosebaceous unit. At the base of the hair bulb is the dermal papilla, whose primary purpose is to connect growing hair with a steady blood supply for nutrient and oxygen delivery as well as waste product removal. The dermal papilla is part of the upper dermis and forms ridges to increase the surface area between the dermis and the surrounding epidermal cells of the hair matrix. The size of the dermal papilla determines the ultimate size of the hair [4].

Surrounding the dermal papilla is the hair matrix, which is composed of specialized germinating epithelial cells. These cells keratinize as they differentiate and move upward to form the centrally located hair shaft. Melanocytes interspersed among the matrix cells produce pigment for the hair shaft [4].

The hair shaft consists of three layers. From deep to superficial, they are the medulla, the cortex, and the cuticle. The medulla contains structural proteins that are different from other keratins and are not well characterized; this layer is absent in vellus hairs. The cortex, which is composed of intermediate filaments and associated proteins, constitutes the bulk of the hair shaft. The cuticle is made up of a single layer of flattened cells [6]. Structurally, the size and shape of the hair shaft may vary between different racial groups. For example, African Americans tend to have more elliptical hair shafts located eccentrically within the hair follicle whereas Asians and Caucasians tend to have more circular hair shafts located centrally within the follicle [4].

Immediately enveloping the hair shaft is the inner root sheath (IRS). The IRS is also composed of three layers: the IRS cuticle, Huxley's layer, and Henle's layer from innermost to outermost. The IRS cuticle is one cell layer thick and interlocks with the hair shaft cuticle to anchor the hair in place and serve as a mold for the growing shaft. Huxley's layer is composed of two or three layers of flattened keratinized cells, and Henle's layer is made up of clear squamous to cuboidal cells. All three concentric layers are characterized by their large eosinophilic cytoplasmic inclusions called trichohyaline granules, which are structural proteins unique to the

IRS and hair follicle medulla [7]. Together, the IRS layers form a mechanically supportive tube for the hair shaft up to the level of the isthmus and seal the lower segment of the pilosebaceous unit from the environment. In the isthmus, proteolytic enzymes degrade the IRS, allowing the hair shaft to emerge from the skin without a surrounding IRS [6] (Fig. 1.1).

TRICHOLOGY TERMS	
Hair (follicle) cycle	Autonomous, rhythmic transformation of fully developed hair follicles through phases of growth, regression and resting; essentially controlled by the follicle itself (by an as yet enigmatic "hair cycle clock"), yet modulated by numerous systemic/extrafollicular factors
Anagen	Growth stage of the hair follicle cycle
Catagen	Involution of the lower two-thirds of the hair follicle by massive keratinocyte apoptosis
Telogen	Resting phase of the hair follicle cycle
Exogen	Phase of active hair shaft shedding (during anagen IV)
Kenogen	Telogen follicle with no club hair present
Hair bulb	Lowermost portion of the hair follicle
Hair matrix	Rapidly proliferating keratinocytes that terminally differentiate to produce the hair shaft
Club hair	Fully keratinized proximal tip of hair shaft, formed during late catagen and telogen; brush-like appearance; characteristic of telogen follicles
Vellus hair (follicle)	Very short, non-pigmented, and usually non-medullated; absence of arrector pili muscle; tiny vellus follicles can display extremely large sebaceous glands (face); undergo full hair cycle, yet much shorter than terminal hair
Terminal hair	Large, usually pigmented and medullated hair
Lanugo hair	Fine hair on the fetal body; shed in utero or during the first weeks of life
Vibrissae	Special sensory hair follicles with unique anatomy and biology, found on the upper lips/snout region of rodent skin, but not in humans; largest and most densely innervated hair follicles with special sinusoid blood supply; first hair follicles to develop
Tylotrich hair follicle	Large sensory hair follicles interspersed within truncal skin, most notably in rodents; extra large, long hair shaft, typically associated with double sebaceous gland and an innervated epidermal Merkel cell complex (Pinkus'Haarscheibe); second type of hair follicle to develop
Non-tylotrich pelage hair	Majority of all hair follicles, last to develop
Effluvium	Excessive shedding of hair shafts (=process)
Alopecia	Abnormal hair loss (=result)
Hirsutism	Excessive vellus-to-terminal hair conversion in androgen-dependent areas in women
Miniaturization	Terminal-to-vellus hair conversion (e.g. on the balding scalp during androgenetic alopecia); these miniaturized follicles still have an arrector pill muscle (unlike true vellus hairs)
Infundibulum of follicle	Region extending from the junction with the interfollicular epidermis to the opening of the sebaceous gland; displays cornification similar to that of the interfollicular epidermis
Isthmus of follicle	Region located between the opening of the sebaceous gland and the site of insertion of the arrector pili muscle; displays trichilemmal keratinization
Arrector pill muscle	Inserts at the level of the bulge; pulls up hair ("goose bumps")
Bulge	Segment of the outer root sheath located at the level of arrector pili muscle insertion; major seat of epithelial stem cells of the hair follicle
Secondary hair germ	Additional seat of epithelial and also of melanocyte stem cells; located between club hair and dermal papilla in telogen hair follicle
Connective tissue sheath (CTS)	Special mesenchymal follicular sheath that is tightly attached to the hair follicle basement membrane and is continuous with the follicular dermal papilla
Follicular dermal papilla (DP)	Onion-shaped, closely packed, specialized fibroblast population with inductive and morphogenic properties; hair cycle-dependent fibroblast trafficking occurs between CTS and DP; volume of DP determines size of hair bulb and, thus, hair shaft diameter
Inner root sheath (IRS)	Packages and guides the hair shaft; cornifies
Outer root sheath (ORS)	Merges distally into the epidermis and proximally into the hair bulb; provides slippage plane, nutrition, regulatory molecules, and stem cells
Follicle pigmentary unit	Melanin-producing hair follicle melanocytes located above and around the upper one-third of the DP; transfer eu- or pheomelanosomes to differentiating hair follicle keratinocytes in the precortical matrix; goes largely into apoptosis during each catagen phase, regenerated from melanocyte stem cells in hair germ (and from non-melanogenic ORS melanocytes?) during anagen

Fig. 1.1 Table of trichology terms. (Modified from Bolognia et al. [17])

Outside of the IRS is the outer root sheath (ORS), also called the trichilemma based on the Greek word meaning "the outer shell around a hair." The ORS is composed of stratified epithelial cells that are continuous with the basal layer of the epidermis. In contrast to cells of the hair shaft and IRS, which move up and out of the hair follicle during growth, cells of the ORS remain stationary. Below the isthmus, ORS cells do not keratinize like IRS cells do. However, at the level of the isthmus when the IRS disintegrates, ORS cells begin to keratinize and accompany the hair follicle up to the epidermis [4].

Importantly, the ORS has a bulge region at the site where the arrector pili muscle attaches. Many multipotent progenitor and stem cells reside in this bulge region and play essential roles in hair follicle regeneration and cycling. In addition, they take part in forming sebaceous glands and healing the epidermis after injury [8]. Consequently, hair ceases to regrow if the ORS bulge region becomes permanently damaged. The ORS also contains melanocytes, Langerhans' cells, and Merkel cells. These cells play vital roles in pigment production, immunologic function, and sensory detection [4].

The outermost layer of the hair follicle is the fibrous root sheath. Composed of thick collagen bundles, it surrounds the entire hair from the dermal papilla up to the papillary dermis. Mesenchymal stem cells in the fibrous root sheath help in dermal wound healing [6].

Hair grows in follicular units, which are naturally occurring groupings of one or more hairs served by one arrector pili muscle and surrounded by a collagen band called the perifolliculum. On average, 10–20% of hair grows as a single follicular unit, 50–60% of hair grows as two-hair follicular units, 10–20% of hair grows as three-hair follicular units, and very few grow as four- or more-hair follicular units [6] (Fig. 1.2).

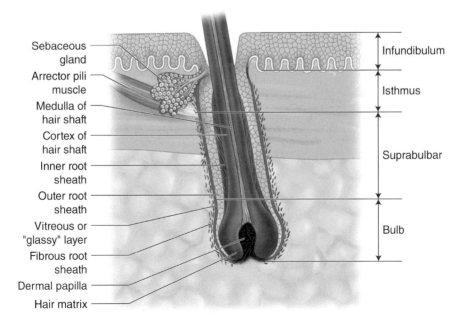

Fig. 1.2 Hair anatomy. (Modified from Demis et al. [18])

Phases of the Hair Cycle

Approximately 5 million hair follicles cover the human body at birth, including about 100,000 on the scalp [6]. No additional hair follicles are regenerated after birth, but each existing follicle continuously cycles through three phases: growth (anagen), regression (catagen), and quiescence (telogen). Hair follicle cycling is self-driven and continues seamlessly even when follicular units are isolated from the skin and grown in culture [9].

Depending on the particular individual, about 85–100% of terminal scalp hair is in the anagen phase at any given time, about 1–2% is in the catagen phase, and about 10–15% is in the telogen phase. The percentage of terminal telogen hair present on the scalp is called the telogen count. This number may be measured with a tricho-gram, phototrichogram, or scalp biopsy. A telogen count greater than 20% is considered abnormal, whereas one between 15% and 20% may require further clinical workup [1]. Different areas of the scalp may also have different standards for what is considered a normal telogen count; specifically, the frontal and vertex regions typically have higher counts compared to other regions [6].

Except for scarring alopecias and rare congenital defects in keratin synthesis, hair loss and undesired hair growth can usually be attributed to abnormalities in the hair cycle. For example, androgenic alopecia may be caused by progressive shortening of the anagen phase while telogen effluvium is characterized by early entry of hair into the telogen phase. Conversely, an overly extended anagen phase may result in conditions such as hirsutism or hypertrichosis [4] (Fig. 1.3).

Anagen

For human terminal scalp hairs, the anagen phase typically lasts 2–3 years, but in some individuals, it may last as long as 7 years. The length of this period is genetically determined and is proportional to the resulting length of hair. Therefore, some individuals who have naturally longer anagen phases can have their hair grow very long, whereas those with shorter anagen phases might not be able to grow their hair beyond a certain length regardless of how long they wait [10].

During anagen, the dermal papilla increases in size and secretes growth factors that signal the surrounding matrix cells to divide rapidly. This process requires a high level of metabolic support, so anagen hairs are particularly sensitive to nutritional deficiencies and chemical injuries such as chemotherapy. As the matrix cells differentiate and migrate upward, they add to the hair shaft at a rate of about 1 cm every 28 days. Notably, this growth rate is unaffected by cutting or shaving of existing hair. Normal anagen hair remains firmly rooted in the scalp and is difficult to remove, except in certain inflammatory conditions of the scalp and diseases like loose anagen syndrome [11]. The hair bulb's degree of axial symmetry during this growth stage determines the overall curvature of the hair. At the end of anagen, fibroblast growth factor 5 and other signaling pathways cause the hair follicle to stop growing and enter the catagen phase [12].

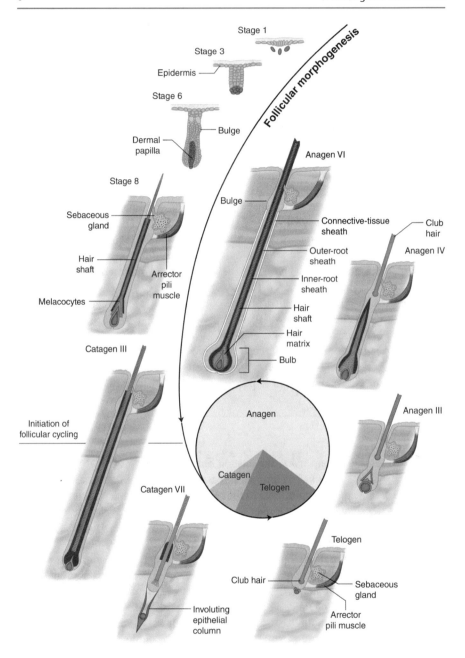

Fig. 1.3 Phases of the hair cycle. (Modified from Paus and Cotsarelis [4]). (Modified from Bolognia et al. [17])

Catagen

Catagen is a brief transitional period that typically lasts between 2 and 3 weeks regardless of hair type or follicle size. This stage is characterized by a significant change in the structure of the hair follicle, the cessation of melanin production in the hair bulb, and the apoptosis of follicular keratinocytes and melanocytes [13].

At the start of catagen, the hair matrix disintegrates and is replaced by a rim of keratinized epithelial cells around the dermal papilla, which reduces in volume by 50% compared to anagen. The remaining precursor hair follicle cells form the base of the hair shaft, called the club fiber, and migrate superficially. This process cuts the hair off from its underlying blood supply. The dermal papilla also begins to disintegrate, condense, and follow the epithelial cells superficially into the dermis, coming to rest just beneath the hair follicle bulge. If the papilla fails to reach this bulge region and interact with bulge stem cells during catagen, the hair follicle stops cycling and is unable to regrow. This phenomenon is seen in individuals with mutations in the *hairless* gene and results in permanent alopecia [14]. At the end of catagen, the hair follicle is about 1/6 of its original length, and everyday activity may dislodge the hair strand [4].

Telogen

Telogen occurs when hair shafts mature into club hairs—fully keratinized, dead hair—that are eventually shed from the follicle. This phase typically lasts 2–3 months. During this time, the club fiber at the base of the telogen hair shaft progressively keratinizes until it occupies approximately the full width of the hair follicle. The club end of the telogen hair also has a surrounding epithelial coating derived from the ORS. At the conclusion of the progressive keratinization, the hair shaft is shed. On any given day, the human scalp loses about 50–150 terminal hairs, with substantial variation between individuals [3]. It remains unclear whether shedding is an actively regulated process or a more passive occurrence where the newly growing hair shaft pushes the old hair out of the follicular canal [15].

During telogen, the bulge region of the ORS is in a resting state and the existing hair shaft does not grow. However, the dermal papilla cells that migrated up to the bulge region during catagen are able to send activating signals through the WNT, SHH, and noggin pathways in order to promote progression to anagen. Changes in the hair follicle environment, such as fluctuations of microRNA levels, have also been shown to induce a change from telogen to anagen [16]. Once the hair germ cells from the bulge are activated by these signals, they expand to form the new hair matrix. The newly growing anagen hair then begins to extend down from the bulge region into the hair bulb and the hair cycle restarts [3].

References

1. Sperling LC, Cowper SE, Knopp EA. An atlas of hair pathology with clinical correlations, second edition. London: CRC Press; 2012.
2. Randall VA. Androgens and hair growth. Dermatol Ther. 2008;21(5):314–28.
3. Bolognia JL, Cerroni L. Dermatology: 2-volume set. Philadelphia: Elsevier; 2017.
4. Paus R, Cotsarelis G. The biology of hair follicles. N Engl J Med. 1999;341(7):491–7.
5. Obana N, Chang C, Uno H. Inhibition of hair growth by testosterone in the presence of dermal papilla cells from the frontal bald scalp of the postpubertal stumptailed macaque. Endocrinology. 1997;138:356–61.
6. Sperling LC. Hair anatomy for the clinician. J Am Acad Dermatol. 1991;25:1–17.
7. Sugiyama S. Cytochemistry of trichohyalin granules: a possible role for cornification of inner root sheath cell in the hair follicle. J Dermatol. 1989;16(2):89–97.
8. Ma DR, Yang EN, Lee ST. A review: the location, molecular characterisation and multipotency of hair follicle epidermal stem cells. Ann Acad Med Singap. 2004;33(6):784–8.
9. Philpott MP, Sanders D, Westgate GE, Kealey T. Human hair growth in vitro: a model for the study of hair follicle biology. J Dermatol Sci. 1994;7(Suppl):S55–72.
10. Braun-Falco O. Dermatology. Heidelberg: Springer Verlag; 2000.
11. Price VH, Gummer CL. Loose anagen syndrome. J Am Acad Dermatol. 1989;20:249–56.
12. Rosenquist TA, Martin GR. Fibroblast growth factor signalling in the hair growth cycle: expression of the fibroblast growth factor receptor and ligand genes in the murine hair follicle. Dev Dyn. 1996;205:379–86.
13. Lindner G, Botchkarev VA, Botchkareva NV, Ling G, van der Veen C, Paus R. Analysis of apoptosis during hair follicle regression. Am J Pathol. 1997;151:1601–17.
14. Ahmad W, Faiyaz ul Haque M, Brancolini V, et al. Alopecia universalis associated with a mutation in the human hairless gene. Science. 1998;279:720–4.
15. Chuong C-M. Molecular basis of epithelial appendage morphogenesis. In: Molecular biology intelligence unit 1. Austin: R.G. Landes; 1998.
16. Mardaryev AN, Ahmed MI, Vlahov NV, et al. Micro-RNA-31 controls hair cycle-associated changes in gene expression programs of the skin and hair follicle. FASEB J. 2010;24(10):3869–81.
17. Bolognia JL, Jorizzo JL, Schaffer JV. Dermatology. Philadelphia: Saunders; 2012.
18. Demis DJ, Thiers BH, Smith EB, et al., editors. Clinical dermatology. Philadelphia: JB Lippincott; 1991. p. 3.

Medical Treatments for Androgenetic Alopecia

2

Dustin H. Marks, Jean-Phillip Okhovat, and Maryanne Makredes Senna

Introduction

Encompassing both male (e.g., male balding) and female pattern hair loss (e.g., female pattern hair thinning), androgenetic alopecia (AGA) represents the most common sub-type of alopecia in the United States, impacting up to 50% of men and women aged 40 years and older [1]. Although numerous shampoos, topical treatments, and oral vitamins and supplements are marketed to the consumer with claims to prevent hair loss and/or promote hair regrowth, there are currently only three FDA-approved medical treatments—topical minoxidil, oral finasteride, and low-level laser therapy—for this type of hair loss. This chapter will accordingly focus on the first-line, FDA-approved therapies for AGA in men and women and additionally review second-line, non-FDA-approved therapies with evidenced-based efficacy as highlighted in Table 2.1.

First-Line, FDA-Approved Medical Treatments for AGA

(a) *Topical Minoxidil:* Topical minoxidil represents the most extensively studied medical treatment for male and female pattern hair loss, demonstrating high efficacy and tolerability in randomized controlled trials.

    (i) Mechanism of Action: Topical minoxidil is available in a 2% solution, 5% solution, or 5% foam and is used in both male and female pattern hair loss. It is thought to promote hair growth by prolonging the anagen (growth)

D. H. Marks · J.-P. Okhovat
Massachusetts General Hospital, Department of Dermatology, Harvard Medical School, Boston, MA, USA

M. M. Senna (✉)
MGH Hair Loss Clinic; Hair Academic Innovative Research (HAIR) Unit, Department of Dermatology, Massachusetts General Hospital, Harvard Medical School, Boston, MA, USA
e-mail: msenna@partners.org

© Springer Nature Switzerland AG 2020
L. N. Lee (ed.), *Hair Transplant Surgery and Platelet Rich Plasma*,
https://doi.org/10.1007/978-3-030-54648-9_2

Table 2.1 Evidence-based treatments for androgenetic alopecia

Treatment	Indication	Evidence-based dosing	Adverse events	Other considerations
FDA approved treatments for AGA				
Finasteride (PO)	MPHL	1 mg QD	Erectile dysfunction, decreased libido, ejaculatory dysfunction, temporary decrease in sperm counts. At higher doses, gynecomastia, testicular pain, and depression	May result in decreased serum PSA levels; should be used in caution in patients with liver dysfunction
Low-level laser therapy (device)	FPHL, MPHL	At least 3–4 times/week; time dependent on device	Temporary itching or tingling of scalp	LLLT bands and helmets may not effectively penetrate the scalp in individuals with darker hair and/or greater hair densities
Minoxidil (topical)	FPHL, MPHL	For FPHL, topical 2% solution BID or topical 5% solution or foam QD; For MPHL, topical 5% solution or foam BID	Contact dermatitis, irritant dermatitis, temporary shedding of hair, scalp pruritus, flaking, facial hypertrichosis	Should not be taken while pregnant or breastfeeding
Non-FDA approved treatments for AGA				
Dutasteride (PO)	MPHL	0.5 mg QD	Erectile dysfunction, decreased libido, ejaculatory dysfunction, temporary decrease in sperm counts, gynecomastia, testicular pain, depression	May result in decreased serum PSA levels; should be used in caution in patients with liver dysfunction
Flutamide (PO)	FPHL	Loading dose of 250 mg QD for year one, followed by 125 mg QD for year two, and 62.5 mg QD for following years	Hepatotoxicity, headaches, respiratory tract disorders, nausea and/or vomiting, diarrhea, dry skin, libido reduction	May consider in women with other sequelae of hyperandrogenism; should not be taken while pregnant or breastfeeding; routine LFT monitoring should be considered

Table 2.1   (continued)

Treatment	Indication	Evidence-based dosing	Adverse events	Other considerations
Ketoconazole (shampoo)	FPHL[a], MPHL	2% KCZ shampoo up to once daily, ensuring that shampoo is left on for 5 minutes	Abnormal hair texture, irritation, increased hair loss, scalp pustules, mild dryness, itching, burning, contact dermatitis, and other application site reactions	Evidence based on men with AGA although may be efficacious in FPHL
Latanoprost (topical)	FPHL[a], MPHL	Topical latanoprost 0.1% solution up to once daily	Scalp erythema, folliculitis, burning, and erysipelas	Evidence based on men with AGA although may be efficacious in FPHL; not commercially available in 0.1% solution
Minoxidil (PO)	FPHL, MPHL	For FPHL, 0.25 mg QD in combination with spironolactone 25 mg QD; For MPHL, 5 mg QD	Hypertrichosis, pedal edema, EKG alterations, postural hypotension, urticaria[b]	Not commercially available in 0.25 mg; should not be taken while pregnant or breastfeeding
Spironolactone (PO)	FPHL	100–200 mg QD	Hyperkalemia and other electrolyte abnormalities, renal dysfunction, gynecomastia, breast tenderness, irregular menses or amenorrhea, postural hypotension, nausea, vomiting, dizziness, and urticaria	May consider in women with other sequelae of hyperandrogenism; should not be taken while pregnant or breastfeeding; should reconcile medication list for potential drug interactions; may consider routine or semi-routine electrolyte monitoring

Abbreviations: *AGA* androgenetic alopecia, *BID* twice a day, *FPHL* female pattern hair loss, *LLLT* low-level laser therapy, *MG* milligrams, *MPHL* male pattern hair loss, *PO* taken by mouth, *QD* once daily
[a]Evidence based on men with AGA although may be efficacious in FPHL
[b]Urticaria suspected to be secondary to spironolactone

phase of hair follicles, shortening the telogen (rest) phase, and enlarging miniaturized hair follicles [2]. Additionally, as a vasodilator, minoxidil works by inducing the production of vascular endothelial growth factor (VEGF), which may help in increasing vascularity and the size of dermal papillae [3, 4].

(ii) Efficacy: In a large randomized trial comparing 2% and 5% minoxidil solution, 393 men (ages 18–49) with androgenetic alopecia were randomly assigned to either 2% topical minoxidil solution ($n = 158$), 5% topical minoxidil solution ($n = 157$), or placebo ($n = 78$) twice daily. Results demonstrated that, after 48 weeks of therapy, 5% minoxidil solution was superior to 2% solution or placebo in terms of increasing nonvellus hair counts (increase of 18.6, 12.7, and 3.9 cm^2, respectively). Additionally, response to treatment occurred earlier with the 5% minoxidil solution as well as improvement in patients' psychosocial perceptions of hair loss [5]. In a later systematic review and meta-analysis of randomized trials for female pattern hair loss, women treated with topical minoxidil (1, 2, or 5%) were significantly more likely to report clinically significant hair regrowth compared to placebo groups (risk ratio 1.93, 95% CI 1.51–2.47) [6]. In a phase III, multicenter, parallel-design clinical trial comparing the efficacy and safety of 5% minoxidil foam versus placebo-vehicle in women with female pattern hair loss, 5% minoxidil topical foam resulted in regrowth of 10.9 hairs/cm^2 and 9.1 hairs/cm^2 at 12 and 24 weeks, respectively, compared to vehicle foam [7].

(iii) Adverse Events: The most common side effects of topical minoxidil include contact dermatitis and irritant dermatitis. Unlike oral minoxidil, topical minoxidil does not alter blood pressure or heart rate, though caution should still be taken in patients with cardiovascular disease due to the potential for systemic absorption [8]. Additionally, shedding of hair can occur in the first 2–8 weeks of treatment, as hairs in the telogen phase are transitioned from telogen to anagen [9]. Other adverse effects can include scalp pruritus, flaking, and facial hypertrichosis; of note, there is a lower risk for scalp irritation with the 5% foam formulation, given the absence of propylene glycol [10].

(iv) Dosing/Administration: Men should apply 1 mL of minoxidil 5% solution or half a capful of 5% foam twice daily to involved areas on a dry scalp. The solution can be spread lightly on the scalp with a finger. Women can apply 1 mL of minoxidil 2% solution twice daily or 1 mL of 5% minoxidil solution once daily or half a capful of 5% foam once daily to affected areas on the scalp. Women should apply the product at least 2 hours before bed to allow the minoxidil to dry and prevent the spread of solution to other parts of the body.

(v) Other Considerations: Although there are no adequate human studies, topical minoxidil has demonstrated adverse effects on the fetus in animal studies. Thus, the use of topical minoxidil is not recommended during pregnancy due to the potential for systemic absorption.

(b) *Oral Finasteride*: Oral finasteride had demonstrated significant utility in the treatment of AGA in men but shown more equivocal results for AGA in women.

(i) Mechanism of Action: Finasteride is a competitive inhibitor of the 5-alpha reductase type 2 enzyme, inhibiting the conversion of testosterone to DHT [11]. At a dose of 1 mg/day, which is typically prescribed for male androgenetic alopecia, finasteride can lower serum and scalp DHT levels by more than 60% [12].

(ii) Efficacy: In two 1-year trials, 1553 men (ages 18–41) with male pattern hair received oral finasteride 1 mg/day or placebo, and 1215 men continued in blinded extension studies for a second year. Efficacy of finasteride treatment was evaluated by scalp hair counts, patient and investigator assessments, and review of photographs by an expert panel. Results demonstrated that finasteride treatment improved scalp hair by all evaluation techniques at 1 and 2 years ($p < 0.001$ vs. placebo). There were clinically significant increases in hair count, measured in a 1-inch diameter circular area of balding vertex scalp, with finasteride treatment (107 and 138 hairs vs placebo at 1 and 2 years, respectively). Additionally, patients' self-assessment showed that finasteride treatment slowed hair loss, increased hair growth, and improved appearance of hair [13]. Studies have additionally shown the efficacy of oral finasteride in males with frontal male pattern hair loss as well. In a 1-year, double-blind, placebo-controlled study, finasteride 1 mg/day resulted in a significant increase in hair count in the frontal scalp of finasteride-treated patients, in addition to significant improvements in patient, investigator, and global photographic assessments [14].

There are only a few studies that have investigated the safety and efficacy of finasteride in women with female pattern hair loss, overall demonstrating variable results. In a 1-year, double-blind, placebo-controlled, randomized, multicenter trial, 137 postmenopausal women (ages 41–60 years) were treated with either finasteride 1 mg/day or placebo. After 1 of therapy, there were no significant differences in the change in hair counts between the finasteride and placebo groups. Furthermore, patient, investigator, photographic assessments, and scalp biopsy analysis did not demonstrate any improvement in slowing hair thinning, increasing hair growth, or improvement in appearance of hair in finasteride versus placebo groups [15]. In another study with 87 normoandrogenic, pre- and post-menopausal women with female pattern hair loss treated with oral finasteride 5 mg/day for 12 months, there were significant increases in hair density and hair thickness, with 70 (81.4%) of 86 patients (1 patient withdrew due to headaches) showing improvements in global photographs [16]. On the other hand, in a randomized, unmasked trial in 36 hyperandrogenic women with alopecia, patients were randomized to either cyproterone acetate (50 mg: *not currently available in the United States*) with ethinyl estradiol in a reverse sequential region, flutamide (250 mg: *discussed later in the chapter*) daily, or finasteride 5 mg daily for 1 year, with 12 similar patients observed without treatment for 1 year. Results demonstrated that flutamide resulted in a reduction of 21% in Ludwig scores, whereas the other treatments—including finasteride—were not statistically significant [17].

(iii) Adverse Events: Reports on the adverse effects of oral finasteride in men have included erectile dysfunction, decreased libido, and ejaculatory dysfunction. In a systematic review of nine trials containing a total of 3570 patients, there was an absolute increase in sexual dysfunction of 1.5% [18]. Furthermore, oral finasteride may result in a temporary decrease in sperm count and production. In one prospective study consisting of 4400 on oral finasteride, semen and hormone parameters were measured before and after discontinuation of finasteride. The mean duration of treatment was 57.4 months and mean dose was 1.04 mg/day. Results demonstrated an average 11.6-fold increase in sperm counts after finasteride discontinuation. Moreover, of men with severe oligospermia (<5 M/mL), 57% had counts increase to normal levels after finasteride cessation. There were no changes in hormone parameters, sperm motility, or sperm morphology after cessation of finasteride [19]. Other rare but potential side effects of oral finasteride may include gynecomastia, testicular pain, and depression, although these side effects are more common on higher doses (5 mg/day) of the medication [20].

(iv) Dosing/Administration: Treatment of male androgenetic alopecia with oral finasteride is recommended at 1 mg/day with or without food. Treatment must be continued for at least 12 months to assess the full effects of the medication and must be taken indefinitely to maintain its efficacy. Oral finasteride is not routinely recommended for female pattern hair loss due to weak evidence supporting its use for this condition.

(v) Other Considerations: It is important to note that oral finasteride can significantly decrease the measurement of serum prostate-specific antigen (PSA). As such, it may theoretically increase the risk for high-grade prostate cancer lesions and all patients' urologists should be notified of the use of this medication [21]. Furthermore, as finasteride is metabolized by the liver, caution should be taken in patients with liver dysfunction.

(c) *Low-Level Laser Therapy*: Low-level laser therapy is effective for both male and female pattern hair loss with randomized controlled trials demonstrating its efficacy compared to sham devices.

(i) Mechanism of Action: Although the exact mechanism of action of low-level laser therapy (LLLT) is unknown, studies have suggested that it may lead to hair regrowth by accelerating mitosis and stimulating hair follicle stem cells or activating follicular keratinocytes [22]. In addition, LLLT has been proposed to alter cell metabolism by disassociating inhibitory nitric oxide from cytochrome c oxidase, leading to increased ATP production and cellular activity [23, 24]. Other studies have also shown LLLT to decrease inflammatory prostaglandin E-2 and other pro-inflammatory cytokines, and to increase anti-inflammatory cytokines such as transforming growth factor-beta 1 and interleukin-10 [25–28].

(ii) Efficacy: In a double-blind, sham device-controlled, multicenter, 26-week trial, 110 male patients with androgenetic alopecia were randomized to treatment with a laser comb (a handheld low-level laser therapy device that contains a single laser module that emulates 9 beams at a wavelength of ~655 nm) or a sham device (2:1). Subjects in the laser comb group demonstrated a significantly greater increase in mean terminal hair density than subjects in the control group ($p < 0.0001$). Additionally, there were significant improvements in overall hair regrowth with respect to patients' subjective assessment at 26 weeks over baseline ($p < 0.015$) [29]. LLLT is equally efficacious for female pattern hair loss. Other randomized trials including patients with male and female pattern hair loss have demonstrated an increase in terminal hair density, and subjects' self-assessment in thickness and fullness of their hair compared to control subjects [30].

(iii) Adverse Events: There are currently no well-established side effects with the use of the laser devices. While some patients may report itching or tingling of their scalp with initial use of the device, this may be due to increased blood flow to the treated areas. As these devices do not emit heat or UV radiation, they do not result in burns to the scalp or increase the risk of skin cancer [31].

(iv) Dosing/Administration: There are currently a variety of models of LLLT on the market. These include a number of laser helmets, bands, combs, and wands. These devices are designed to be used three times a week to achieve desirable results with specific time requirements for each device ranging from 3 to 15 minutes per treatment [31].

(v) Other considerations: Increased hair density and/or darker hair may impact penetration of the LLLT to the scalp; in such cases, use of a comb or other handheld device may be more beneficial in such patients to ensure adequate penetration to the scalp. Another consideration is the difficulty of use of a comb or wand with patients with shoulder and other musculoskeletal issues affecting range of motion; in such cases, handless devices may be more suitable.

Second-Line, Non-FDA-Approved Medical Treatments for AGA

(a) *Dutasteride*: Dutasteride is a potent inhibitor of type 1 and type 2 5-alpha-reductase that has demonstrated efficacy for male pattern hair loss in randomized controlled trials.

(i) Mechanism of Action: Dutasteride is an inhibitor of both type 1 and type 2 5-alpha-reductase and is a much more potent inhibitor of the enzyme than finasteride. For instance, serum levels of DHT can lower by as much as 93–94% at a dose of 0.5 mg/day of dutasteride, compared to 70% at a dose of 5 mg/day of finasteride [32].

(ii) Efficacy: In a randomized, placebo-controlled trial of 416 men (ages 21–45), patients were randomized to receive either dutasteride 0.05 mg/day, dutasteride 0.1 mg/day, dutasteride 0.5 mg/day, dutasteride 2.5 mg/day, finasteride 5 mg/day, or placebo daily for 24 weeks. Results demonstrated an increase in target area hair count versus placebo in a dose-dependent fashion with dutasteride 2.5 mg/day superior to finasteride at 12 and 24 weeks. Results were confirmed by expert panel photographic review and investigator assessment of hair growth. Additionally, scalp and serum DHT levels decreased, whereas testosterone levels increased, in a dose-dependent manner on the various doses of dutasteride. However, 13% of men on the dutasteride 2.5 mg/day dose reported decreased libido [33]. In another randomized, double-blind phase III study comparing the efficacy, safety, and tolerability of dutasteride in male pattern hair loss, 153 men (ages 18–49) were randomized to receive either 0.5 mg dutasteride or placebo daily for 6 months. Results demonstrated a mean increase of hair counts of $12.2/cm^2$ in the dutasteride group compared to $4.7/cm^2$ in the control group ($p = 0.0319$); these results were supported by subject self-assessment and investigator and panel photographic assessment [34]. There are no well-established randomized controlled trials to demonstrate the efficacy of dutasteride for female pattern hair loss.

(iii) Adverse Events: As a more potent inhibitor of type 1 and type 2 5-alpha-reductase, dutasteride may have a similar although less tolerable side effect profile as finasteride. These include erectile dysfunction, decreased libido, ejaculatory dysfunction, a temporary decrease in sperm count, gynecomastia, testicular pain, and depression.

(iv) Dosing/Administration: Although dutasteride is not routinely prescribed for male pattern hair loss, it is sometimes prescribed off-label at a dose of 0.5 mg/day for male androgenetic alopecia.

(v) Other Considerations: Similar to finasteride, caution must be taken when interpreting PSA levels as dutasteride may lower PSA levels and thus lower potential suspicion for prostate carcinoma.

(b) *Flutamide*: Limited prospective studies have demonstrated moderate efficacy of oral flutamide for the treatment of FPHL [17, 35, 36].

(i) Mechanism of Action: Flutamide represents a selective nonsteroidal anti-androgenic agent without other hormonal or antihormonal properties. It functions largely at the peripheral level, selectively blocking the cytoplasmic and nuclear binding of androgens [35]. Its primary FDA-approved indication is for the treatment of metastatic prostate carcinoma in men; however, it has also displayed some utility in managing signs and symptoms of hyperandrogonism in women [37].

(ii) Efficacy: In the largest cohort to date, a prospective study of 101 women with FPHL, the women were treated with flutamide for 4 years [35]. Participating women received a tapering regimen of flutamide with a loading dose of 250 mg/day for the first year, 125 mg/day for the second year, and 62.5 mg/day for the third and fourth years. Furthermore, the majority (68 out of 101, 67%) received flutamide in combination with an oral contraceptive pill (OCP), while a minority (33 out of 101, 33%) received flutamide alone. A significant improvement ($p < 0.001$) in Ludwig scores was observed after 6 months of treatment and continued to improve over the next 2 years until stabilizing. No significant difference was observed between flutamide with and without an oral contraceptive with mean improvement in Ludwig scores of 15%, 20%, 26%, and 28% at 0.5, 1, 1.5, and 2 years, respectively [35]. A smaller prospective cohort of 12 hyperandrogenic women found that daily flutamide 250 mg for 1 year resulted in a small but significant ($P < 0.05$) reduction in average Ludwig scores of 21% from 2.3 at the start of treatment to 1.8 following 1 year of treatment [17]. Of note, an earlier randomized controlled trial (RCT)—which primarily investigated the treatment of hirsutism—found that 6 months of flutamide at 250 mg BID in combination with an OCP increased "cosmetically acceptable hair density" in 6 of 7 women with AGA. No changes in alopecia were noted in the comparison arm of Spironolactone at 50 mg BID [36].

(iii) Adverse Events: In the aforementioned prospective cohort study of 101 women, 4 (4.0%) patients displayed transaminitis during daily dosing of 250 mg. After treatment was discontinued, all labs demonstrated normal transaminase values. Other mild and temporary adverse events reported in the cohort included headaches (5.9%), respiratory tract disorders (4.0%), nausea and/or vomiting (5.0%) diarrhea (3.0%), dry skin (8.9%), and libido reduction (5.0%) [35].

(iv) Dosing/Administration: Currently, there is no standard dosing regimen for oral flutamide treatment for FPHL. Given that transient transaminitis was observed at once-daily dosing of 250 mg, clinicians should take caution when prescribing higher dosing regimens of flutamide and may consider more routine lab monitoring [35].

(v) Other Considerations: While there are no controlled data in human pregnancy, flutamide has demonstrated teratogenic effects in offspring born to female rats treated during late pregnancy and thus should not be considered for FPHL during pregnancy [38]. Given its anti-androgenic properties, this medication should also not be considered for MPHL. Additionally, clinicians may monitor liver function tests given the potential of hepatoxicity. However, there is currently no evidenced-based standard or recommendation on lab monitoring for women taking flutamide.

(c) *Ketoconazole*: A small comparative, prospective study demonstrated equivalent efficacy of daily 2% ketoconazole (KCZ) shampoo and daily 2% minoxidil lotion for MPHL [39].

(i) Mechanism of Action: KCZ represents an imidazole broad-spectrum antifungal and biosynthesis inhibitor [40]. The shampoo form currently serves as the gold standard for treating mild to moderate dandruff and seborrheic dermatitis via a dualistic mechanism of reducing both *Malassezia* colonization and surrounding inflammation. Separately, it has also been proposed that AGA may result, at least in part, from the presence of lipophilic microorganisms in the hair follicle unit that trigger an inflammatory and immunoregulatory response and subsequently contribute to the hair loss. Thus, KCZ shampoo therapeutic mechanism of action in the treatment of AGA may be comparable to its role in seborrheic dermatitis with direct anti-inflammatory impact and reduction of microorganisms on the scalp [39]. Additionally, ketoconazole has also exhibited androgen-lowering potential and can potentially inhibit dihydrotestosterone production and/or dihydrotestosterone binding to androgen receptors [40].

(ii) Efficacy: In a two-part comparative study, Pierard-Franchimont et al. [39] first investigated the use of 2% KCZ shampoo compared to unmedicated shampoo in 39 men with grade III vertex AGA according to the Hamilton–Norwood scale. After the use of the control or experimental shampoo for 2–4 times weekly over a 21-month period, the KCZ group, in comparison to the control group, displayed a progressive increase in AGA pilary index (PI, proportion of anagen hairs × average diameter). The PI increase in the KCZ group was evident after 6-months and reached a plateau value after 15 months (~2000 PI at 1 month versus 3750 PI at 15 months). A linear regression model comparing KCZ PI and time was significant ($r = 0.69$, $p < 0.01$). Given these results, the investigators then followed two groups of four men with grade III vertex AGA for 6 months using daily 2% KCZ shampoo or the combination of 2% minoxidil lotion and unmedicated shampoo wash. After 6 months of treatment, both the KCZ and minoxidil groups showed improvement in hair density (+18% and +11%, respectively) and median hair shaft diameter (+7%, +7%). Furthermore, a decrease in the sebaceous gland area was demonstrated in the KCZ group (−19.4%) in comparison to an increase seen in the minoxidil group (+5.3%) [39].

(iii) Adverse Events: In 264 patients using 2% KCZ shampoo for dandruff and/or seborrheic dermatitis treatment, <1% developed increased hair loss and irritation. Other reported adverse events include abnormal hair texture, scalp pustules, mild dryness, itching, burning, contact dermatitis, and other application site reactions [41].

(iv) Dosing/Administration: Patients should be instructed to apply the shampoo to a damp scalp, lather, leave in place for 5 minutes, and then rinse off up to once a day [41].

(v) Other Considerations: Although no controlled studies have been reported to date, 2% KCZ shampoo may also be considered for FPHL as the proposed mechanism should also apply to women with AGA.

(d) *Latanoprost*: A randomized, double-blind placebo-controlled study supported the use of topical latanoprost 0.1% solution for AGA [42].

(i) Mechanism of Action: Primarily indicated for open-angle glaucoma and ocular hypertension as an ophthalmic solution (0.005%) and more recently used to stimulate eyelash growth, latanoprost functions as a prostaglandin F2α (PGF2α) analog. Based on murine and other animal models, it is supported that PGF2α promotes hair regrowth and melanogenesis by increasing vasodilation in the dermis and inducing DNA replication and cell division in addition to influencing the role of keratinocytes, dermal fibroblasts, and mast cells which may promote the anagen growth phase [43].

(ii) Efficacy: The highest-grade evidence for topical latanoprost 0.1% solution for AGA results from a double-blind, randomized study of 16 male participants with grade II–III frontotemporal alopecia according to the

Hamilton–Norwood scale [42]. Two 3 cm^2 minizones of alopecia on each patient were randomly assigned to treatment with latanoprost or control solution. After 24 weeks of daily use, latanoprost-treated sites displayed significantly higher increases ($P < 0.001$) in hair densities (+22%) when compared to placebo and baseline, according to TrichoScan data. In comparison, there was no significant difference in the anagen/telogen ratio from baseline to 24 weeks, although the absolute number of both anagen (115–127 hairs/cm^2) and telogen (64–90,115–127 hairs/cm^2) hairs increased [42].

(iii) Adverse Events: In the aforementioned proof of concept study, 8 out of 16 (50%) subjects displayed an adverse event to topical latanoprost including scalp erythema ($n = 5$), folliculitis ($n = 1$), burning ($n = 1$), and erysipelas ($n = 1$) over the 24 week study period [42]. The 0.005% ophthalmic solution has also been associated with iris pigment and eyelid skin darkening, eyelash changes, and macular edema [44]. However, these reported adverse effects are associated with repeated exposure directed at the eye which would not be indicated for use in AGA.

(iv) Dosing/Administration: Currently, latanoprost solution is commercially available only as 0.005% ophthalmic solution thus requiring special pharmacy compounding at the higher dose demonstrated for hair loss. In the pilot study, an investigational product of 0.1% ternary solution (50% ethanol, 20% propylene glycol, water) was created and subsequently packed into 50 μL droppers for daily use on a 3 cm^2 area [42].

(v) Other Considerations: As mentioned earlier, the 0.1% solution is not commercially available and thus will require a special compounding pharmacy and potentially result in higher out of pocket costs. Additionally, similar to KCZ shampoo, no controlled studies have been reported on latanoprost solution for women with FPHL. Although the proposed mechanism should be equally efficacious in men and women, there is currently no evidence of its treatment in FPHL. Of final considerations, another prostaglandin analog, bimatoprost 0.03% solution, was trialed in one patient with FPHL via injections but was not shown to be efficacious [45].

(e) *Oral Minoxidil*: While topical minoxidil has been extensively studied for AGA and accordingly represents one of three FDA-approved treatments for this indication, limited, non-comparative case series and cohorts have supported the use of oral minoxidil as monotherapy for MPHL and in combination with oral spironolactone for FPHL [46, 47].

(i) Mechanism of Action: Please refer to the earlier discussion on topical minoxidil.

(ii) Efficacy: In the first report to determine the efficacy and safety of oral minoxidil for AGA, 30 men with grade III to V vertex AGA according to the Hamilton–Norwood scale received oral minoxidil 5 mg daily for 24 weeks. After the 24-week study period, oral minoxidil significantly increased total hair counts at the vertex from baseline to 26.0 hairs/cm^2 (14.25%) at 12 weeks to 35.1 26.0 hairs/cm^2 (19.23%) at 24 weeks

($p = 0.007$). The frontal hairline also demonstrated a significant response but to a lesser degree than the vertex. Additionally, based on global photography using a 7-point rating scale, 43% of patients demonstrated a score improvement of +3 [46]. More recently, a prospective, uncontrolled, open-label observational study of 100 women with Sinclair stage 2-5 FPHL reported on a combination therapy of once-daily minoxidil 0.25 mg and spironolactone 25 mg. After 6 and 12 months of therapy, the mean reduction in hair loss severity score was 0.85 and 1.3, respectively. There was also a mean reduction in hair shedding score from 2.3 at 6 months to 2.6 at 12 months. Based on these preliminary results, the authors argued that combination therapy of minoxidil 0.25 mg and spironolactone 25 mg are safe and effective treatments of FPHL but further placebo-controlled studies are necessary [47].

   (iii) Adverse Events: At lower doses, oral minoxidil is generally well tolerated but higher doses (e.g., 5 mg+) used for severe hypertension may result in a more extensive adverse event profile. In the cohort study of 30 men with AGA receiving oral minoxidil 5 mg daily, adverse events included hypertrichosis ($n = 28$, 93%), pedal edema ($n = 3$, 10%), and EKG alterations (e.g., occasional PVC and T wave change in 1 lead; $n = 3$, 10%) [46]. In comparison, out of 100 women with AGA receiving combination daily oral minoxidil 0.25 mg and spironolactone 25 mg, 8 developed adverse events including urticaria ($n = 2$, 2%), postural hypotension ($n = 2$, 2%), and facial hypertrichosis ($n = 4$, 4%). The urticaria, moreover, was assumed to be related to the spironolactone and when oral minoxidil was continued as monotherapy, the urticaria did not recur. Also of note, 22 patients (22%) reported that a temporary increase in hair shedding at treatment initiation was of substantial concern although no patient discontinued treatment for this reason [47].

   (iv) Dosing/Administration: The current evidence has demonstrated the efficacy of oral minoxidil as monotherapy at 5 mg daily for MPHL and at 0.25 mg daily in combination with spironolactone 25 mg for FPHL.

   (v) Other Considerations: Oral minoxidil tablets are currently available in the United States as 2.5 and 10 mg, thus requiring special compounding into the 0.25 mg dosing that has been reported for use in FPHL. Given the risk of fluid retention with oral minoxidil, especially at higher dosing, spironolactone combination therapy is a reasonable option in FPHL both to mitigate any potential edema and to add an antiandrogen therapeutic mechanism [47]. Women should additionally not take oral minoxidil when pregnant or breastfeeding [48].

(f) *Spironolactone*: Spironolactone has demonstrated utility in the treatment of FPHL although there is still a paucity of prospective, placebo-controlled studies to support its use [49–51].

   (i) Mechanism of Action: Initially indicated as a potassium-sparing diuretic to treat hypertension and later discovered to have utility in the treatment of hirsutism, acne, seborrhea, and polycystic ovarian syndrome (PCOS), spironolactone functions as an aldosterone antagonist with antiandrogenic activity by decreasing both the production and binding of androgens on target tissues. Its antiandrogen properties, furthermore, are more selective to tissue with elevated levels of 17a-hydroxylase and thus substantially reduce 17-hydroxylation of steroids [51].

(ii) Efficacy: In addition to a number of case reports and series, two larger studies have supported the use of spironolactone for FPHL. In the first open, prospective intervention study, 40 women with biopsy-proven FPHL received spironolactone 200 mg daily. The investigation included an additional 40 women receiving cyproterone acetate, an antiandrogen medication that is not commercially available in the United States. After a minimum of 12 weeks, there was no significant difference between spironolactone and cyproterone acetate treatment arms so the authors reported combined results detailing that 44% ($n = 35$) had hair regrowth, 44% ($n = 35$) had no clear change, and 12% ($n = 10$) had continued hair loss [49]. More recently, a combined study included 19 patients with FPHL on spironolactone (mean dose = 110 mg daily) with follow-up ranging from 7 to 20 months from a retrospective review in addition to 20 patients from a survey study. Combing the data, 74.3% of patients ($n = 29$) reported stabilization or improvement of their FPHL since starting spironolactone. Approximately half ($n = 20$, 51%) of the patients demonstrated mild improvement and/or increased thickness [50].

(iii) Adverse Events: At lower doses, spironolactone is generally well tolerated but does exhibit adverse events in a dose-dependent response [51]. The most serious adverse events of this medication include hyperkalemia and renal dysfunction (including renal failure). To mitigate the potential development or worsening of hyperkalemia, patients should avoid frequent and/or large consumptions of potassium-rich foods and supplements in addition to medications that may also increase potassium levels (e.g., ACE inhibitors). Other adverse events include but are not limited to other fluid and electrolyte abnormalities, gynecomastia, breast tenderness, irregular menses or amenorrhea, postural hypotension, nausea, vomiting, dizziness, and urticaria [52].

(iv) Dosing/Administration: Standard, off-label dosing of spironolactone for FPHL is 100–200 mg daily [51]. A limited quantitative assessment of six Caucasian females found that low dose of 75–100 mg/day stabilized FPHL from further progression but initial dosing >150 mg daily may be required to improve hair density [53]. To maximize tolerability, one may consider starting 50 mg daily for 1–2 weeks and titrating upward as needed.

(v) Other Considerations: There are several important considerations to recognize when prescribing spironolactone. Firstly, it has the potential to adversely affect the sex differentiation of the male during embryogenesis and subsequently feminize male fetuses. Consequently, women should not take spironolactone when pregnant or breastfeeding [52]. Secondly, in order to minimize the potential for electrolyte abnormalities and orthostatic hypotension, clinicians should take a detailed history of the patient's medications and note potential drug interactions with ACE inhibitors, barbiturates, narcotics, corticosteroids, skeletal muscle relaxants, lithium, digoxin, and NSAIDs [52]. There is accordingly currently no standard recommendation on routine lab work to monitor for electrolyte abnormalities. Lastly, given its efficacy in treating other signs and symptoms of hyperandrogenism, spironolactone may serve a dual or triple purpose in women with FPHL and concomitant acne, hirsutism, and/or PCOS [51].

Considerations of Oral Contraceptives for Female AGA

(a) In patients with female pattern hair loss, oral contraceptive pills (OCPs) should additionally be considered as they may either paradoxically treat or promote further hair loss. Combined oral contraceptive pills (COCs), more specifically, contain both estrogen and progesterone components. While the included estrogen is typically ethinyl estradiol at variable doses, the progesterone component varies widely [54]. Largely categorized as testosterone derivatives or androgen receptor antagonists, the progestins available in COCs have demonstrated unique androgenicity based on the specific chemical structure [54, 55]. Accordingly, progestins associated with lower androgenicity should be considered for patients with FPHL as they may protect against further hair loss, while progestins associated with higher androgenicity should be avoided. Of the progestins available in current COCs, drospirenone, ethynodiol diacetate, norethindrone, and norethindrone acetate have demonstrated the lowest androgen index (equal to the product of progestin androgenicity and cumulative monthly dose) [56]. Notably, there is a paucity of literature investigating the androgenicity of COCs in the clinical setting and head-to-head comparisons of their impact on the hair cycle. Until further evidence is obtained, clinicians may recommend a monophasic COC with a regular to a high dose of estrogen (>30 mcg) and a third- or fourth-generation progesterone (e.g., Ocella, Kelnor, Balziva). Before starting or switching COCs, patients should be appropriately counseled on the associated increased risks of venous thromboembolism, pulmonary embolism, stroke, some cancers, and—of particular relevance to this patient population—telogen effluvium [54].

Considerations of Vitamins and Mineral Supplements for AGA

(a) In general, recommendations regarding routine use of micronutrient supplements should be approached with caution as the US Food and Drug Administration (FDA) is not required to review safety or efficacy profiles of vitamins and minerals supplements prior to marketing, and compliance with Good Manufacturing Practice regulations remains substandard [57]. Except for patients with increased requirements, proper nutrient intake can be achieved through a well-balanced diet as micronutrients in food are usually better absorbed and associated with fewer adverse effects than supplements [57, 58]. These principles, furthermore, should similarly be followed for all patients with AGA. In some cases, patients, especially reproductive-aged women, may benefit from iron supplementation for their hair loss. Of the other numerous available vitamins and mineral supplements advertised to promote hair growth and health, a novel nutraceutical product containing a proprietary Synergen Complex® has displayed the most promising, evidence-based efficacy [59]. In contrast, biotin supplementation should not be recommended to treat AGA given its limited utility and potential to interfere with critical lab tests [60–62].

(b) *Iron*: Representing the most commonly deficient nutrient in the world, iron is an essential cofactor for ribonucleotide reductase, the rate-limiting step in DNA synthesis. Iron, therefore, plays a critical role within the hair follicular unit and other tissues with high cellular turnover [63]. Moreover, the relationship between iron deficiency and numerous types of hair loss has been investigated. While there are currently no evidence-based recommendations, all patients presenting with hair loss may be screened for iron deficiency as a treatment for AGA may be optimized when iron deficiency, regardless of anemia status, is treated [64]. Of all the iron markers, serum ferritin has the greatest predictive value for true iron status and thus represents the most useful test when determining iron deficiency. More specifically, the lower limit cut-off value of 41 ng/mL provides a sensitivity and specificity of 98% for iron deficiency [64]. Using a comparable cut-off value of 40 ng/mL, a prospective study investigated the use of cyproterone acetate-ethinyl estradiol for FPHL and found that patients with serum ferritin concentrations >40 ng/mL experienced more significant increases in mean total and meaningful hair densities ($P < 0.01$) than patients with serum ferritin <40 ng/mL [65]. Accordingly, patients with AGA may be screened for iron deficiency using serum ferritin levels. Individuals with serum ferritin <40 ng/mL may subsequently be started on a once-daily iron supplement to maximize the efficacy of other first- and second-line, evidenced-based treatments.

(c) *Nutraceutical Supplement*: While numerous vitamins and mineral supplements are marketed to improve hair quantity and/or quality, the greater majority is not supported by evidenced-based claims. In comparison, a randomized, double-blind, placebo-controlled study evaluated a nutraceutical supplement (Nutrafol®) that contains a number of active botanical ingredients (e.g., Ashwagandha, Biocurcumin, Saw Palmetto, and vitamin E) with potential anti-inflammatory, antioxidant, and dihydrotestosterone-inhibiting properties. Although the study was limited by number with 40 subjects in total, the nutraceutical supplement significantly increased the number of terminal and vellus hairs and overall hair quality ($p < 0.05$) in women with self-perceived thinning hair [59]. As it remains unregulated by the FDA and demonstrated efficacy in one small RCT, this supplement should not be recommended as the first-line treatment for AGA. However, in patients specifically requesting to include a vitamin or supplement in their treatment regimen for AGA, Nutrafol® may be considered after the discussion on its limited regulations.

(d) *Biotin*: Biotin, otherwise known as Vitamin B7 or Vitamin H, represents a water-soluble B vitamin that is necessary for the cellular metabolism of fatty and amino acids and gluconeogenesis. To date, no clinical trials have surveyed its efficacy in the treatment of any form of hair loss despite its ubiquity in social media and direct-to-consumer advertisements for this indication [62, 66]. A comprehensive review of the literature, moreover, concluded that there is an overarching lack of clinical evidence to support the use of biotin to improve hair quantity and/or quality. Accordingly, biotin should not be routinely recommended as a treatment for AGA [66]. In fact, the FDA recently released a safety communication addressing the potential dangers of biotin as high levels can cause significant incorrect lab test results [60]. Case reports and series have revealed that high-dose biotin consumption may lead to a falsely low TSH level and elevated free T4 (lab markers routinely assessed in patients with alopecia) and of greater concern, falsely low troponin tests which resulted in the death of one patient with a misdiagnosed myocardial infection [60–62]. Consequently, for patients already taking biotin for hair loss, it should be recommended to discontinue this vitamin given its lack of efficacy for hair loss treatment and the greater potential to interfere with critical lab tests.

Final Recommendations and Considerations

(a) Recommendations for MPHL: While oral finasteride represents a more potent treatment, topical minoxidil 5% foam or solution applied twice daily should be considered as the first-line treatment for MPHL. If the patient subsequently desires more aggressive medical intervention, oral finasteride 1 mg may be recommended. However, thorough counseling with patients should be provided especially to younger men who may theoretically take the systemic medication for decades.

(b) Recommendations for FPHL: Although there is an even greater paucity of randomized, placebo-controlled trials of hair loss treatments for FPHL in comparison to MPHL, topical minoxidil 5% foam or solution applied once daily should be considered as a first-line treatment. For women with hormone-induced acne, hirsutism, or PCOS or those requiring additional medical intervention, spironolactone 50 mg twice daily may be considered.

(c) General considerations for all medical treatments for androgenetic alopecia: Regardless of the medical treatment started for hair loss, it should be continued for at least 6–12 months before an objective improvement can be observed as hair grows at the rate of approximately 1 cm/month. Furthermore, any hair loss treatment that is initiated must be continued indefinitely to sustain utility. Termination of any efficacious treatment will result in the loss of regrown or preserved hair within months.

References

1. Otberg N, Shapiro J. Chapter 88. Hair growth disorders. In: Fitzpatrick's dermatology in general medicine, 8e | AccessMedicine | McGraw-Hill Medical [Internet]. 8th ed. New York: The McGraw-Hill Companies; 2012. [cited 6 Sep 2018]. Available from: https://accessmedicine-mhmedical-com.ezp-prod1.hul.harvard.edu/Content.aspx?bookId=392&sectionId=41138795.
2. Messenger AG, Rundegren J. Minoxidil: mechanisms of action on hair growth. Br J Dermatol. 2004;150:186–94.
3. Lachgar S, Charveron M, Gall Y, Bonafe JL. Minoxidil upregulates the expression of vascular endothelial growth factor in human hair dermal papilla cells. Br J Dermatol. 1998;138:407–11.
4. Li M, Marubayashi A, Nakaya Y, Fukui K, Arase S. Minoxidil-induced hair growth is mediated by adenosine in cultured dermal papilla cells: possible involvement of sulfonylurea receptor 2B as a target of minoxidil. J Invest Dermatol. 2001;117:1594–600.
5. Olsen EA, Dunlap FE, Funicella T, Koperski JA, Swinehart JM, Tschen EH, et al. A randomized clinical trial of 5% topical minoxidil versus 2% topical minoxidil and placebo in the treatment of androgenetic alopecia in men. J Am Acad Dermatol. 2002;47:377–85.
6. van Zuuren EJ, Fedorowicz Z, Schoones J. Interventions for female pattern hair loss. Cochrane Database Syst Rev. 2016;(5):CD007628.
7. Bergfeld W, Washenik K, Callender V, Zhang P, Quiza C, Doshi U, et al. A phase III, multi-center, parallel-design clinical trial to compare the efficacy and safety of 5% minoxidil foam versus vehicle in women with female pattern hair loss. J Drugs Dermatol. 2016;15:874–81.
8. Ebner H, Müller E. Allergic contact dermatitis from minoxidil. Contact Dermatitis. 1995;32:316–7.
9. Blumeyer A, Tosti A, Messenger A, Reygagne P, Del Marmol V, Spuls PI, et al. Evidence-based (S3) guideline for the treatment of androgenetic alopecia in women and in men. J Dtsch Dermatol Ges. 2011;9(Suppl 6):S1–57.
10. Olsen EA, Messenger AG, Shapiro J, Bergfeld WF, Hordinsky MK, Roberts JL, et al. Evaluation and treatment of male and female pattern hair loss. J Am Acad Dermatol. 2005;52:301–11.
11. Rittmaster RS. Finasteride. N Engl J Med. 1994;330:120–5.
12. Price VH. Treatment of hair loss. N Engl J Med. 1999;341:964–73.
13. Kaufman KD, Olsen EA, Whiting D, Savin R, DeVillez R, Bergfeld W, et al. Finasteride in the treatment of men with androgenetic alopecia. Finasteride Male Pattern Hair Loss Study Group. J Am Acad Dermatol. 1998;39:578–89.
14. Leyden J, Dunlap F, Miller B, Winters P, Lebwohl M, Hecker D, et al. Finasteride in the treatment of men with frontal male pattern hair loss. J Am Acad Dermatol. 1999;40:930–7.
15. Price VH, Roberts JL, Hordinsky M, Olsen EA, Savin R, Bergfeld W, et al. Lack of efficacy of finasteride in postmenopausal women with androgenetic alopecia. J Am Acad Dermatol. 2000;43:768–76.
16. Yeon JH, Jung JY, Choi JW, Kim BJ, Youn SW, Park KC, et al. 5 mg/day finasteride treatment for normoandrogenic Asian women with female pattern hair loss. J Eur Acad Dermatol Venereol. 2011;25:211–4.
17. Carmina E, Lobo RA. Treatment of hyperandrogenic alopecia in women. Fertil Steril. 2003;79:91–5.
18. Mella JM, Perret MC, Manzotti M, Catalano HN, Guyatt G. Efficacy and safety of finasteride therapy for androgenetic alopecia: a systematic review. Arch Dermatol. 2010;146:1141–50.
19. Samplaski MK, Lo K, Grober E, Jarvi K. Finasteride use in the male infertility population: effects on semen and hormone parameters. Fertil Steril. 2013;100:1542–6.
20. Rahimi-Ardabili B, Pourandarjani R, Habibollahi P, Mualeki A. Finasteride induced depression: a prospective study. BMC Clin Pharmacol. 2006;6:7.
21. D'Amico AV, Roehrborn CG. Effect of 1 mg/day finasteride on concentrations of serum prostate-specific antigen in men with androgenic alopecia: a randomised controlled trial. Lancet Oncol. 2007;8:21–5.

22. Lubart R, Eichler M, Lavi R, Friedman H, Shainberg A. Low-energy laser irradiation promotes cellular redox activity. Photomed Laser Surg. 2005;23:3–9.
23. Eells JT, Wong-Riley MTT, VerHoeve J, Henry M, Buchman EV, Kane MP, et al. Mitochondrial signal transduction in accelerated wound and retinal healing by near-infrared light therapy. Mitochondrion. 2004;4:559–67.
24. Pastore D, Greco M, Passarella S. Specific helium-neon laser sensitivity of the purified cytochrome c oxidase. Int J Radiat Biol. 2000;76:863–70.
25. Arany PR, Nayak RS, Hallikerimath S, Limaye AM, Kale AD, Kondaiah P. Activation of latent TGF-beta1 by low-power laser in vitro correlates with increased TGF-beta1 levels in laser-enhanced oral wound healing. Wound Repair Regen. 2007;15:866–74.
26. de Lima FM, Villaverde AB, Albertini R, Corrêa JC, Carvalho RLP, Munin E, et al. Dual effect of low-level laser therapy (LLLT) on the acute lung inflammation induced by intestinal ischemia and reperfusion: action on anti- and pro-inflammatory cytokines. Lasers Surg Med. 2011;43:410–20.
27. Mafra de Lima F, Villaverde AB, Salgado MA, Castro-Faria-Neto HC, Munin E, Albertini R, et al. Low intensity laser therapy (LILT) in vivo acts on the neutrophils recruitment and chemokines/cytokines levels in a model of acute pulmonary inflammation induced by aerosol of lipopolysaccharide from Escherichia coli in rat. J Photochem Photobiol B. 2010;101:271–8.
28. Sakurai Y, Yamaguchi M, Abiko Y. Inhibitory effect of low-level laser irradiation on LPS-stimulated prostaglandin E2 production and cyclooxygenase-2 in human gingival fibroblasts. Eur J Oral Sci. 2000;108:29–34.
29. Leavitt M, Charles G, Heyman E, Michaels D. HairMax LaserComb laser phototherapy device in the treatment of male androgenetic alopecia: a randomized, double-blind, sham device-controlled, multicentre trial. Clin Drug Investig. 2009;29:283–92.
30. Jimenez JJ, Wikramanayake TC, Bergfeld W, Hordinsky M, Hickman JG, Hamblin MR, et al. Efficacy and safety of a low-level laser device in the treatment of male and female pattern hair loss: a multicenter, randomized, sham device-controlled, double-blind study. Am J Clin Dermatol. 2014;15:115–27.
31. Frequently Asked Questions [Internet]. HairMax. Available from: https://hairmax.com/pages/faq-1.
32. Amory JK, Wang C, Swerdloff RS, Anawalt BD, Matsumoto AM, Bremner WJ, et al. The effect of 5alpha-reductase inhibition with dutasteride and finasteride on semen parameters and serum hormones in healthy men. J Clin Endocrinol Metab. 2007;92:1659–65.
33. Olsen EA, Hordinsky M, Whiting D, Stough D, Hobbs S, Ellis ML, et al. The importance of dual 5alpha-reductase inhibition in the treatment of male pattern hair loss: results of a randomized placebo-controlled study of dutasteride versus finasteride. J Am Acad Dermatol. 2006;55:1014–23.
34. Eun HC, Kwon OS, Yeon JH, Shin HS, Kim BY, Ro BI, et al. Efficacy, safety, and tolerability of dutasteride 0.5 mg once daily in male patients with male pattern hair loss: a randomized, double-blind, placebo-controlled, phase III study. J Am Acad Dermatol. 2010;63:252–8.
35. Paradisi R, Porcu E, Fabbri R, Seracchioli R, Battaglia C, Venturoli S. Prospective cohort study on the effects and tolerability of flutamide in patients with female pattern hair loss. Ann Pharmacother. 2011;45:469–75.
36. Cusan L, Dupont A, Gomez JL, Tremblay RR, Labrie F. Comparison of flutamide and spironolactone in the treatment of hirsutism: a randomized controlled trial. Fertil Steril. 1994;61:281–7.
37. Euflex (flutamide 250 mg tablets) package insert from Merck Canada Inc. [Internet]. 2011. Available from: https://hemonc.org/docs/packageinsert/flutamide.pdf.
38. Goto K, Koizumi K, Takaori H, Fujii Y, Furuyama Y, Saika O, et al. Effects of flutamide on sex maturation and behavior of offspring born to female rats treated during late pregnancy. J Toxicol Sci. 2004;29:517–34.
39. Piérard-Franchimont C, De Doncker P, Cauwenbergh G, Piérard GE. Ketoconazole shampoo: effect of long-term use in androgenic alopecia. Dermatology. 1998;196:474–7.
40. Hugo Perez BS. Ketocazole as an adjunct to finasteride in the treatment of androgenetic alopecia in men. Med Hypotheses. 2004;62:112–5.

41. NIZORAL® (KETOCONAZOLE) 2% SHAMPOO package insert from Janssen Pharmaceuticals [Internet]. 2013. Available from: https://www.accessdata.fda.gov/drugsatfda_docs/label/2013/019927s032lbl.pdf.

42. Blume-Peytavi U, Lönnfors S, Hillmann K, Garcia Bartels N. A randomized double-blind placebo-controlled pilot study to assess the efficacy of a 24-week topical treatment by latanoprost 0.1% on hair growth and pigmentation in healthy volunteers with androgenetic alopecia. J Am Acad Dermatol. 2012;66:794–800.

43. Sasaki S, Hozumi Y, Kondo S. Influence of prostaglandin F2α and its analogues on hair regrowth and follicular melanogenesis in a murine model. Exp Dermatol. 2005;14:323–8.

44. Xalatan® latanoprost ophthalmic solution 0.005% (50 µg/mL) package insert from Pfizer Inc [Internet]. 2011. Available from: https://www.accessdata.fda.gov/drugsatfda_docs/label/2012/020597s044lbl.pdf.

45. Emer JJ, Stevenson ML, Markowitz O. Novel treatment of female-pattern androgenetic alopecia with injected bimatoprost 0.03% solution. J Drugs Dermatol. 2011;10:795–8.

46. Lueangarun S, Panchapreteep R, Tempark T, Noppakun N. Efficacy and safety of oral minoxidil 5 mg daily during 24-week treatment in male androgenetic alopecia. J Am Acad Dermatol. 2015;72:AB113.

47. Sinclair RD. Female pattern hair loss: a pilot study investigating combination therapy with low-dose oral minoxidil and spironolactone. Int J Dermatol. 2018;57:104–9.

48. Loniten® minoxidil tablets, USP package insert from Pfizer Inc [Internet]. 2015. Available from: https://www.accessdata.fda.gov/drugsatfda_docs/label/2015/018154s026lbl.pdf.

49. Sinclair R, Wewerinke M, Jolley D. Treatment of female pattern hair loss with oral antiandrogens. Br J Dermatol. 2005;152:466–73.

50. Shannon F, Christa S, Lewei D, Carolyn G. Demographics of women with female pattern hair loss and the effectiveness of spironolactone therapy. J Am Acad Dermatol. 2015;73:705–6.

51. Rathnayake D, Sinclair R. Innovative use of spironolactone as an antiandrogen in the treatment of female pattern hair loss. Dermatol Clin. 2010;28:611–8.

52. Aldactone® spironolactone tablets, USP package insert by Pfizer Inc [Internet]. 2008. Available from: https://www.accessdata.fda.gov/drugsatfda_docs/label/2008/012151s062lbl.pdf.

53. Rushton DH, Futterweit W, Kingsley D, Kinglsey P, Norris M. Quantitative assessment of spironolactone treatment in women with diffuse androgen-dependent alopecia. J Soc Cosmet Chem. 1991;42:317–25.

54. Azarchi S, Bienenfeld A, Lo Sicco K, Marchbein S, Shapiro J, Nagler AR. Androgens in women: hormone modulating therapies for skin disease (part II). J Am Acad Dermatol. 2018;80:1509.

55. Carr BR. Uniqueness of oral contraceptive progestins. Contraception. 1998;58:23S–7S.

56. Ho A, Shapiro J, Sukhdeo K. Ranking oral contraceptives for pattern hair loss: use of the androgen index (abstract). 2018.

57. Manson JE, Bassuk SS. Vitamin and mineral supplements: what clinicians need to know. JAMA. 2018;319:859–60.

58. Rautiainen S, Manson JE, Lichtenstein AH, Sesso HD. Dietary supplements and disease prevention – a global overview. Nat Rev Endocrinol. 2016;12:407–20.

59. Ablon G, Kogan SA. Six-month, randomized, double-blind, placebo-controlled study evaluating the safety and efficacy of a nutraceutical supplement for promoting hair growth in women with self-perceived thinning hair. J Drugs Dermatol. 2018;17:558–65.

60. The FDA warns that biotin may interfere with lab tests: FDA safety communication [Internet]. US Food Drug Adm. 2017. Available from: https://www.fda.gov/medicaldevices/safety/alertsandnotices/ucm586505.htm.

61. Ardabilygazir A, Afshariyamchlou S, Mir D, Sachmechi I. Effect of high-dose biotin on thyroid function tests: case report and literature review. Cureus. 2018;10:e2845.

62. Lipner SR. Rethinking biotin therapy for hair, nail, and skin disorders. J Am Acad Dermatol. 2018;78:1236–8.

63. Thompson JM, Mirza MA, Park MK, Qureshi AA, Cho E. The role of micronutrients in alopecia areata: a review. Am J Clin Dermatol. 2017;18:663–79.

64. Trost LB, Bergfeld WF, Calogeras E. The diagnosis and treatment of iron deficiency and its potential relationship to hair loss. J Am Acad Dermatol. 2006;54:824–44.
65. Rushton DH, Ramsay ID. The importance of adequate serum ferritin levels during oral cyproterone acetate and ethinyl oestradiol treatment of diffuse androgen-dependent alopecia in women. Clin Endocrinol. 1992;36:421–7.
66. Soleymani T, Lo Sicco K, Shapiro J. The infatuation with biotin supplementation: is there truth behind its rising popularity? A comparative analysis of clinical efficacy versus social popularity. J Drugs Dermatol. 2017;16:496–500.

Hair Loss Physiology and Transplantation Principles

3

Tymon Tai, Michael S. Chow, and Amit Kochhar

Hair Loss Physiology

Pathophysiology

In the healthy scalp, hair is replenished commensurate with the rate at which hair is lost, resulting in a cosmetically stable hair pattern. In male and female patterned hair loss, two major disruptions to this equilibrium take place: hair cycle perturbation and follicular miniaturization. Androgen-driven alteration of the hair cycle truncates the anagen phase, which can effectively shorten total hair length until hair shafts no longer reach the surface of the skin. During the catagen/telogen phase, which is protracted in patterned hair loss, the follicular units miniaturize and form into thin vellus hairs from thick pigmented terminal hairs. The ratio of terminal to vellus hair also decreases, further contributing to the appearance of balding [1].

Endocrinologically, testosterone and its derivatives are the primary drivers of male patterned hair loss. Circulating testosterone exerts its effects by directly binding to androgen receptors (AR) on the cells of the dermal papilla (DPC) or by 5-alpha reductase-mediated conversion into dihydrotestosterone (DHT), which has a fivefold increase in binding affinity for AR [2]. Of the two 5-alpha reductase types, type II is typically concentrated within DPCs and more involved in hair loss.

T. Tai
Keck School of Medicine of USC, USC Caruso Department of Otolaryngology Head and Neck Surgery, Los Angeles, CA, USA

M. S. Chow
New York University, Department of Otolaryngology – Head and Neck Surgery, New York, NY, USA

A. Kochhar (✉)
Facial Plastic and Reconstructive Surgery, Pacific Neuroscience Institute, Santa Monica, CA, USA
e-mail: Amit.kochhar@med.usc.edu

© Springer Nature Switzerland AG 2020
L. N. Lee (ed.), *Hair Transplant Surgery and Platelet Rich Plasma*,
https://doi.org/10.1007/978-3-030-54648-9_3

Manipulation of these pathways forms the basis of pharmacologic alopecia treatment. As mentioned in Chap. 1, the effects of androgen binding depend on scalp location. The follicles of the beard, axilla, and pubis increase in size when subject to androgen binding, while the follicles of the frontal scalp and vertex undergo miniaturization. The occipital and temporal scalp is spared as its follicles are largely unaffected by androgen activity. Different embryologic origins are suspected to account for these discrepancies – frontoparietal scalp dermis forms from neural crest cells while occipital and temporal scalp originates from mesoderm [1]. Modern hair transplantation leverages this phenomenon of site specificity as androgen-independent hair follicles are transplanted to areas of baldness.

While the major mechanisms in male pattern hair loss are understood, the causes of female pattern hair loss require further study as there are significant biochemical differences between sexes. For example, the female scalp possesses cytochrome p450 aromatase, which competitively converts testosterone into estradiol and estrone over DHT, in addition to lowering 5-alpha reductase levels [3]. It is therefore suspected that female pattern hair loss operates through androgen-independent pathways.

Phenotypes of Patterned Hair Loss

The site-specific and sex-dependent nature of androgen binding to DPCs usually manifests as a typical balding pattern. The Ludwig classification system characterizes female pattern baldness, in which the frontal hairline is usually unaffected but rather a generalized thinning and increasing middle part forms. This middle part is often characterized as a "Christmas tree" pattern (Fig. 3.1) [4]. In males, it is

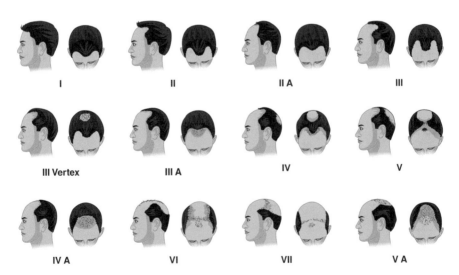

Fig. 3.1 Norwood classification of male pattern hair loss. The Norwood classification system stratifies male patients into seven stages of severity. As balding progresses, the frontotemporal hairline shifts from a convex to a concave shape and the vertex becomes increasingly involved

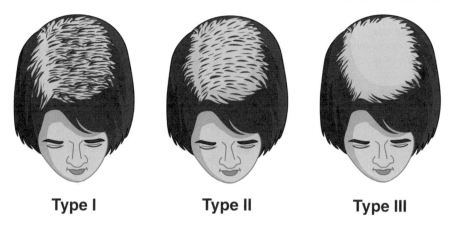

Type I   **Type II**   **Type III**

Fig. 3.2 Ludwig classification of female pattern hair loss. The Ludwig classification system stratifies female patients into three stages of alopecia. In addition to a generalized thinning, hair loss in the middle part becomes more accentuated. This pattern is sometimes referred to as a "Christmas tree" for its characteristic appearance

frequently described by the Norwood classification system, allowing the surgeon to communicate the degree of vertex thinning and hairline frontotemporal recession as the hairline changes from a concave to convex shape (Fig. 3.2) [5].

Principles of Transplantation

Donor Site Dominance and Site Selection

Successful transplantation of hair follicles from the donor site requires that hair extracted from a healthy scalp donor site will retain its characteristics such as anagen phase duration and remain viable even if it is relocated to an area that can no longer grow hair. This ability of the donor site hair to maintain dominance of its physical traits over the recipient area is called donor site dominance theory [6, 7]. As such, ideal donor follicles should be androgen-insensitive, as donor follicles from androgen-sensitive areas will eventually miniaturize and shed in the same manner than if the follicle had not been transplanted. The quality and location of the donor follicles are important to consider, as hair from different areas of the body will differ in length, texture, strength, pigmentation, etc. A general "safe zone" for donor site selection often presents itself in patients with class V, VI, and VII balding patterns in the occipital region. A good rule of thumb is to place the superior boundary of the donor site at least 2 cm below where crown thinning is predicted to occur and the inferior boundary 2 cm above the nape of the neck – avoiding androgen-sensitive follicles in the superior boundary and the naturally thinning hair of the lower occiput (Fig. 3.3) [8]. The implication here is that the demarcated safe zone is indicative of the patient's final balding pattern. However, it is important to

Fig. 3.3 Identification of a safe donor area. Demarcation of safe donor area boundaries

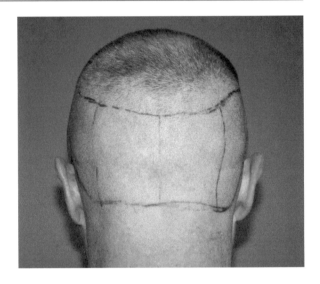

understand that hair loss is a dynamic process and that patients may continue to lose hair beyond the time of consultation. Furthermore, surgeons now understand that terminal hair has the potential to transition into vellus hair decades later after the onset of balding, potentially creating a pattern much different from what was expected. Therefore, it is the surgeon's responsibility to form appropriate patient expectations during consultation and to select a donor site that anticipates and accounts for this potential outcome.

Optimizing for Transplant Success

Success with transplantation of hair follicles relies on principles akin to that of any other tissue graft used in reconstructive surgery. Like skin grafts and other local flaps, several factors must be optimal to achieve successful transplantation including:

1. Limiting graft handling and trauma
2. Limiting graft ischemia time
3. Storage of follicles in nutrition-rich media while awaiting implantation
4. Ensuring an adequate host vascular supply
5. Proper graft placement

Trauma

Physical damage to the follicle can reduce transplanted hair integrity and viability. Follicles are susceptible to transection, crush, and dehydration injury. For this reason, the use of loupes/microscopic magnification is highly recommended when handling donor follicles.

Vascular Supply

As with any graft, a rich vascular bed with adequate oxygenation is critical for graft survival. Variability in scalp oxygenation may be most significant determinant of surgical outcome [9]. Despite a robust vascular supply, diffusion-mediated oxygenation of the scalp can be compromised in patients with medical comorbidities. Scar tissue from inflammatory conditions, trauma, radiation exposure, previous surgery, tobacco use, and chronic illnesses such as diabetes can impair oxygenation. Therefore, the exact transplant density for maximum follicular viability varies. To this end, many therapies aim to improve oxygenation potential. Angiogenic agents (platelet-rich plasma and porcine urinary bladder matrix) and exogenous ATP have been suggested as potential means to overcome inadequate perfusion [10].

Incision depth has also been implicated as a factor in graft survival. Surgeons should aim to place transplanted follicles as close to the natural hair follicle depth as possible. Too superficial and the graft and the bulb may desiccate from inadequate perfusion. Too deep and a surgeon risks damaging other structures (such as blood vessels) and compromising overlying tissue viability.

Metabolic Factors

Numerous biomechanical factors contribute to graft success. Like other transplant procedures, intra-operative graft ischemia time needs to be taken into consideration: once removed from the donor site the follicle has a limited oxygen and nutrient supply. After that supply is exhausted, insufficient energy production via anaerobic metabolism will eventually lead to apoptosis of follicular cells, and even death of the entire follicle. Similarly, follicular grafts are susceptible to reperfusion injury, the phenomenon in which ischemic tissue, when suddenly re-exposed to oxygen after ischemia, forms radical oxygen species (ROS) and that irreversibly damage cells despite restoration of an adequate blood supply [9].

Follicle Storage

Prior to implantation, harvested follicles must be stored in an adequate medium as the recipient site is prepared. Many options for graft storage during ischemia time exist, designed to maintain osmotic balance, buffer pH, and provide nutrients to the harvested follicles. Research demonstrates greatly increased cell viability on a multitude of cell types over the course of a few days in storage solution [11]. However, the choice of medium is often debated, with many surgeons opting to use normal saline or lactated ringers. With commercial storage solutions, the surgeon should understand the optimal concentrations and temperatures for their chosen medium. Use of these solutions outside of their recommended conditions can be detrimental to graft health.

Postoperative Factors

Transplanted follicles can sometimes become disrupted in the postoperative period. Although discussed in greater detail in Chap. 9, education on proper postoperative care is essential to surgical success as seemingly benign scenarios such as excessive washing, hat wearing, and exercise can impair healing.

Summary

Understanding the pathophysiology of pattern baldness, the importance of patient selection, setting appropriate expectations, and surgical planning are all major components of achieving a satisfactory outcome. In male pattern baldness, hair follicles respond to DHT binding, undergoing follicle miniaturization and progressive shortening of the anagen growth phase, resulting in a characteristic pattern. Female pattern hair loss similarly results in a distinct pattern, although the mechanisms for this pathology are less clear. Understanding donor dominance theory and how it affects donor site selection in addition to controlling operative variables is important for the hair surgeon.

References

1. Banka N, Bunagan MJ, Shapiro J. Pattern hair loss in men: diagnosis and medical treatment. Dermatol Clin. 2013;31(1):129–40.
2. Kaufman KD. Androgens and alopecia. Mol Cell Endocrinol. 2002;198(1–2):89–95.
3. Sawaya ME, Price VH. Different levels of 5alpha-reductase type I and II, aromatase, and androgen receptor in hair follicles of women and men with androgenetic alopecia. J Invest Dermatol. 1997;109(3):296–300.
4. Ludwig E. Classification of the types of androgenetic alopecia (common baldness) occurring in the female sex. Br J Dermatol. 1977;97(3):247–54.
5. Norwood OT. Male pattern baldness: classification and incidence. South Med J. 1975;68(11):1359–65.
6. Orentreich N. Autografts in alopecias and other selected dermatological conditions. Ann N Y Acad Sci. 1959;83:463–79.
7. Dinh HV, Sinclair RD, Martinick J. Donor site dominance in action: transplanted hairs retain their original pigmentation long term. Dermatol Surg. 2008;34(8):1108–11.
8. Yun SS, Park JH, Na YC. Hair diameter variation in different vertical regions of the occipital safe donor area. Arch Plast Surg. 2017;44(4):332–6.
9. Cooley JE. Optimal graft growth. Facial Plast Surg Clin North Am. 2013;21(3):449–55.
10. Uebel CO, da Silva JB, Cantarelli D, Martins P. The role of platelet plasma growth factors in male pattern baldness surgery. Plast Reconstr Surg. 2006;118(6):1458–66; discussion 67.
11. Parsley WM, Perez-Meza D. Review of factors affecting the growth and survival of follicular grafts. J Cutan Aesthet Surg. 2010;3(2):69–75.

Indications and Contraindications for Hair Transplant

4

Tymon Tai, Michael S. Chow, Sahar Nadimi, and Amit Kochhar

Health Utility of Hair Transplantation

The objective of this chapter is to aid in the identification of factors that will affect the outcome of hair treatment and to highlight conditions that may make patients appropriate or poor candidates. Consultation of the hair transplant (HT) patient begins with a thorough and open discussion of the patients' concerns and goals for treatment. Despite the benign effects of alopecia on physical health, hair loss patients can suffer significant psychosocial distress including decreased self-esteem, decreased satisfaction with their self-image, and decreased sexual quality of life [1, 2]. This distress may manifest in depressive symptoms and less frequent social engagement [3–5]. Experiments on the perceptions of alopecia also indicate that balding patients are more likely to be rated by others as less attractive, likable, and successful compared to non-balding peers, underscoring potential difficulties with finding romantic relationships and employment [6–8].

In a recent health utility study by Abt et al., adult observers were asked to determine the health states of patients with different conditions including alopecia and

T. Tai
Keck School of Medicine of USC, USC Caruso Department of Otolaryngology Head and Neck Surgery, Los Angeles, CA, USA

M. S. Chow
New York University, Department of Otolaryngology – Head and Neck Surgery, New York, NY, USA

S. Nadimi
Department of Otolaryngology-Head and Neck Surgery, Loyola University Medical Center, Maywood, IL, USA

A. Kochhar (✉)
Keck Hospital of USC School of Medicine, Division of Facial Plastic and Reconstructive Surgery, Department of Otolaryngology, Head and Neck Surgery, Los Angeles, CA, USA

© Springer Nature Switzerland AG 2020
L. N. Lee (ed.), *Hair Transplant Surgery and Platelet Rich Plasma*,
https://doi.org/10.1007/978-3-030-54648-9_4

how much time or risk they would be willing to incur in order to treat said condition [9]. Responses demonstrate that participants would be willing to trade in 7–9% of their remaining life years for a permanent hair loss cure and that the distress posed by alopecia is comparable to that of medium-grade facial paralysis or unilateral deafness with microtia. The desire to correct alopecia was significant enough that subjects were willing to undertake the level of risk incurred in surgery, nearly comparable to that of correction of monocular blindness. Yet, despite the non-trivial effects of this disease, patients often are unsatisfied with their pursuit for non-medical solutions prior to evaluation by a hair surgeon [10]. With this in mind, the surgical consultation should aid the patient to garner a realistic understanding of what they may gain from a successful hair transplant.

Although the literature on the quality of life for alopecia patients is clear about the impact on self-image, there is a paucity of quality of life data for posttransplant patients. A randomized-controlled survey study by Bater et al. demonstrated that alopecia patients were considered more attractive, successful, and approachable after hair transplant [11]. The aforementioned work by Abt et al. went further, illustrating that hair transplant patients were perceived by participants as healthier than balding counterparts based on standard health utility scales [9]. Based on these findings, we can infer that hair transplant does in fact improve perceptions of the balding patient – a benefit that patients should be made aware of.

Indications

Dr. Konior and Simmons summarized the consultation of the surgical hair patient best, noting that "almost every [patient] is a candidate for a hair transplantation provided [they] accept the limitations of surgery and understand the final hair loss pattern that will result." This statement not only emphasizes the finite nature of donor follicles to transplant but also how important it is that the patient maintain realistic expectations throughout the dynamic and potentially decades-long balding process [12]. Patients expecting a complete return to their previous appearance will inevitably be dissatisfied with their surgical outcome. Careful explanation of the procedure's limitations and skillful management of expectations are keys to patient satisfaction. If a patient is unable to accept the realities of this procedure, the transplant should not be performed. Patients with rapidly evolving hairlines should also consider the benefits of watchful waiting until they reach a stable new plateau of hair growth. Similarly, patients need to understand that as the balding process continues and their face ages, a hairline that may seem appropriate at the moment may appear artificial and unsightly in the future. The possibility of subsequent procedures may also be necessary if the hair loss develops further. There is little downside to a more conservative step-wise approach.

Young patients experiencing alopecia are particularly susceptible to forming unrealistic expectations. These patients undergoing hairline regression are accustomed to a full head of hair in addition to an environment of peers who are unfamiliar with or intolerant of balding. These factors may pressure the patient to pursue an aggressive restoration of their hairline. However, the patient's hairline will continue to mature and hair loss will likely continue in some fashion. In time, the graft may thin and potential future donor sites become less available. In conjunction with an aggressive restoration approach, the final outcome when the patient is older may appear synthetic and unflattering. Therefore, candid counseling with this cohort of patients is especially important and may take multiple discussions.

Ideal candidates for hair transplant are patients with treatment goals appropriate for their condition and their facial structure even as they age, patients with a healthy donor site containing sufficient donor hair to create a natural pattern even as hair loss evolves, and patients with a healthy recipient site. In that light, a predictable progression of hair loss allows a surgeon to more confidently identify an area in which hair is unaffected by follicle miniaturization. Other qualities of the donor scalp and hair such as increased thickness and darker pigmentation also contribute to a successful cosmetic outcome. Lastly, transplantation is often part of a larger treatment plan. Adjuvant medical therapy such as minoxidil, finasteride, and platelet-rich plasma can play a role in the treatment of patterned baldness. Insight into a patient's ability to adhere to adjuvant medical therapy and to perform attentive post-operative care is essential to achieving the desired outcome.

Contraindications

Certain conditions can predispose to suboptimal transplant outcomes, in addition to unrealistic expectations on the part of the patient. Others conditions may self-resolve, eliminating the need for a long-term hair restoration plan. The following section covers relative contraindications for transplant candidacy.

Unpatterned or Diffuse Loss

In unpatterned or diffuse hair loss, the surgeon is often unable to predict which area of the scalp will be subject to donor miniaturization, reducing the reliability of the donor site for transplantation.

The most common instances of diffuse hair loss are attributable to telogen effluvium and anagen effluvium. Telogen effluvium is a diffuse thinning of hair in response to physiological or psychological stress: multiple hair follicles simultaneously enter telogen phase resulting in cosmetically appreciable hair loss. General anesthesia, rapid weight loss, pregnancy, and prolonged illness are all possible triggering events [13]. This condition usually self-resolves and rarely requires treatment.

Anagen effluvium is a similar pathology involving loss of hair in the growth phase. This is usually the result of a systemic insult, impairing follicular mitotic, or metabolic activity. The now-weakened hair shaft is prone to fracture upon exiting the skin. Chemotherapy and radiotherapy are the most commonly implicated causes for anagen effluvium. Alopecia secondary to radiation exhibits a dose-response relationship. Patients with none-to-minimal alopecia were found to have received a mean dosage of 32.9 Gy (range 10.7–54.0 Gy) and those with moderate-to-severe alopecia exposed to a mean of 48.4 Gy (range 15.9–73.6 Gy) [14]. In rare cases, anagen effluvium has been observed as a symptom of alopecia areata (AA) and pemphigus vulgaris. Other causes of anagen effluvium include pressure, trauma, radiation, and chemical exposure. The effects are usually reversible with regrowth of hair beginning several weeks after correction of the underlying etiology.

Inflammatory and Cicatricial Conditions

Scarring and inflammatory scalp conditions present similar challenges for the hair transplant surgeon and often represent the same underlying etiology at different time points. Inflammatory conditions such as scarring alopecia, or psoriasis can occur sporadically and present at unpredictable locations on the scalp. The unpredictable nature of these flare-ups can lead to the loss of transplanted follicles or new areas of hair loss post-transplantation.

Fibrosis is a frequent consequence of chronic or extreme inflammation. Scarring of the affected areas can lead to decreased viability of the affected tissue. These areas are at high risk for hypoxia and graft failure.

Autoimmune Conditions

Alopecia Areata

Direct damage of hair follicles by host immunity is termed alopecia areata (AA), leading to patches of circular or ovoid hair loss from the body, face, or scalp. Keratin deposits that appear as yellow dots may be observed (Fig. 4.1). Regrowing hair in the area may undergo poliosis or whitening of the hairshaft. AA is classified based upon the pattern or location of hair loss. This patchy hair loss should not be confused with alopecia totalis, the loss of all hair on the scalp or alopecia universalis, the loss of all hair on the body. As an autoimmune pathology, topical steroids are the mainstay of treatment with most patients experiencing hair regrowth after treatment.

AA is a difficult condition to manage from the hair transplantation perspective. As autoimmune flares can strike at any location involving transplanted hairs, donor hairs or transplanted follicles, it is essential to inform patients of the risk of hair loss unrelated to their procedure if transplantation is pursued.

Diffuse AA or alocepia areata incognita is a rare form of rapid hair loss that is seen predominantly in young women. Due to its fast onset, AA is commonly mistaken for telogen effluvium, but differs in that AA hair follicles can often be easily pulled out and exhibit an "exclamation point" morphology. Patients may endorse early signs of tingling and pruritis to affected areas before hair loss begins.

Lichen Planopilaris

Lichen planopilaris (LPP) differs from AA in that the entire pilosebaceous unit is the target of host autoimmunity. During the active stages of disease, perifollicular

Fig. 4.1 Alopecia areata.
(a) This patient suffers
from severe advanced
alopecia areata with total
scalp hair loss and sparing
of the eyebrows and
eyelashes. (b)
Dermatoscopy of the
patient's scalp,
demonstrating the classic
appearance of yellow
keratin deposits

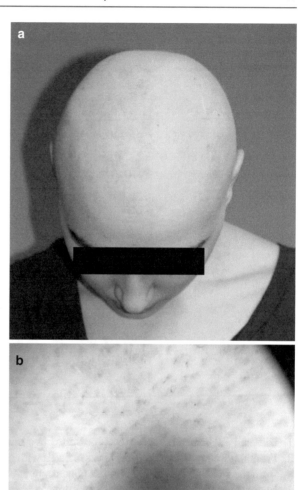

Fig. 4.1 Alopecia areata. (a) This patient suffers from severe advanced alopecia areata with total scalp hair loss and sparing of the eyebrows and eyelashes. (b) Dermatoscopy of the patient's scalp, demonstrating the classic appearance of yellow keratin deposits

erythema can be seen in association with itching or burning sensations. As the disease progresses, patients often experience hair loss resulting in a shiny bald patch (Fig. 4.2). Intervention during the active stage is aimed toward reducing inflammation and minimizing follicle destruction. First line therapy is topical steroidal treatment. In recalcitrant disease, injected or systemic steroids can be considered.

There are three subtypes of LPP (Classic, Frontal Fibrosing, and Lasseur Grahham-Little Piccardi syndrome) which are based upon the pattern and location of hair loss.

Fig. 4.2 Lichen planopilaris. This patient with lichen planopilaris demonstrates a distinct balding patch in the midline scalp

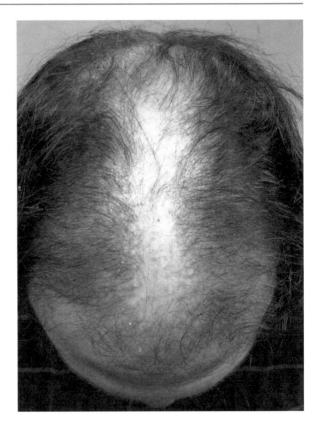

1. Classic LPP preferentially affects the vertex in a multifocal pattern.
2. Frontal fibrosing alopecia (FFA) is associated with progressive scarring hair loss from the frontotemporal region with concurrent eyebrow loss.
3. Lasseur Grahham–Little Piccardi syndrome is characterized by scarring alopecia of the scalp, follicular keratotic papules on glabrous skin of the palms and soles, and variable alopecia of the axillae and groin.

The role for hair transplantation remains unclear. A recent systematic review of 13 articles by Lee et al. found that 29% of patients with FFA and 75% with LLP achieved positive post-transplant results [15]. Despite a nonstatistically significant difference in success rates and a small sample size, the study suggests that certain patients can benefit from HT. Further investigation is necessary to better define this cohort.

Other Autoimmune Conditions
Other etiologies of unpatterned hair loss include generalized autoimmune **processes** such as psoriasis, and discoid lupus erythematosus (DLE). Psoriasis is a dermatologic condition in which the inflammatory cascade is activated in the dermis with hyperactivation of keratinocytes and overproduction of epidermal cells. Extensor surfaces are preferentially affected but in psoriatic alopecia, the scalp is also

involved. Hair usually regrows but instances of scarring alopecia secondary to psoriatic plaques that limits regrowth have been reported. Patients with psoriasis have also been found to be at higher risk for AA.

DLE is a form of chronic cutaneous lupus erythematosus that presents as cutaneous scaly erythematous or violaceous plaques causing significant follicular plugging and subsequent scarring/atrophy. It may occur in conjunction with systemic lupus erythematosus or in the absence of systemic disease. Management of active lesions and minimizing scarring is the cornerstone of treatment. Lesions are most often managed with topical or intralesional corticosteroids. Avoidance of direct sun exposure is also essential to prevent flares.

One controversial diagnosis of cicatricial alopecia is Brocq pseudopelade. In this disorder, hair loss resembles AA but actually represents an endpoint for many different forms of cicatricial alopecia. Hair loss can be focal or widespread with episodic and unpredictable results. Progression is often slow and sporadic but may also rapidly progress. Dermatologists consider this entity a diagnosis of exclusion.

Infectious

Infectious etiologies less frequently cause alopecia but are of fungal origin when present. Tinea capitis occurs as diffuse hair loss secondary to a superficial fungal infection. The presentation is variable: skin can be seen with a non-inflammatory scale reminiscent of seborrheic dermatitis or skin can appear severely inflamed with kerion (deep abscesses). In severe instances, the risk of scarring and permanent alopecia is increased. Diagnosis is obtained by staining of hair and scale from the affected area with potassium hydroxide. Treatment involves oral antifungals and selenium sulfide shampoo with an indication for a short course of steroid if kerions are appreciated.

Psychological/Self-Inflicted

Psychological illness or traumatic habits are a common cause of non-physiologic hair loss that the surgeon should be mindful of during the consultation process. Careful attention to patient habits and patterns of hair loss is helpful to prevent recurrent hair loss even after transplantation.

Trichotillomania, an impulse control disorder in which a patient has urges to pull out their own hair, is the most frequent cause of psychological hair loss. Onset usually occurs in a patient's youth and often coincides with diagnosis of a concomitant personality disorder or anxiety. Symptoms wax and wane with a mean illness duration of 21.9 years, where only 27.3% of patients ultimately seek psychiatric treatment [16]. Patients may not disclose hair-pulling behaviors for fear of social consequences. If no hair-pulling is noted during a patient interview, broken hairs of variable length contained in a circular pattern (friar-tuck sign) and regrowing hair at variable lengths can hint toward self-inflicted hair loss [17]. Treatment includes psychiatric consultation and is rooted in behavioral modification. Most patients will experience regrowth once plucking has discontinued. However, some do experience thinning or balding after extensive trauma to the hair roots. Thorough evaluation for hair-pulling behavior is essential, as a hair transplant procedure is not indicated for these patients. If permanent hair loss is noted and a procedure is pursued, it is essential that the patient has developed appropriate behavioral impulse control. Otherwise, patients who still act on their compulsions, risk trauma to the transplanted follicles and graft failure.

Though trichotillomania is the only psychological diagnosis that results in direct hair trauma, other psychological factors play an important role in candidate selection. The presence of co-morbid psychological diagnoses such as depressive or anxiety disorders can impair the patient's ability to rationally assess the severity of their condition and to form reasonable expectations.

Traction alopecia is hair loss due to inadvertent traumatic habits such as prolonged physical traction on hair shafts from hair styling (e.g., tight buns and braids). The pattern of hair loss is determined by the areas of greatest tension. The majority of patients experience reversal of hair loss after cessation of said traumatic practices.

Summary

Achieving success in follicular transplantation is a multifactorial endeavor. Identification of the patient's hair loss etiology is essential to appropriate surgical planning. A hair transplant surgeon must recognize unpatterned hair loss or any inflammatory, infectious, or psychological sources of alopecia through a thorough history and physical examination. If concern arises for any of these pathologies, a biopsy and referral to respective consultants should be considered without hesitation. Avoidance of procedures with questionable benefit and proper patient selection is equally important as operative acumen. Familiarity with the possibilities and limits of follicular graft transplantation combined with appropriate patient counseling will optimize outcomes.

References

1. Williamson D, Gonzalez M, Finlay AY. The effect of hair loss on quality of life. J Eur Acad Dermatol Venereol. 2001;15(2):137–9.
2. Li SJ, Huang KP, Joyce C, Mostaghimi A. The impact of alopecia areata on sexual quality of life. Int J Trichol. 2018;10(6):271–4.
3. Alfonso M, Richter-Appelt H, Tosti A, Viera MS, Garcia M. The psychosocial impact of hair loss among men: a multinational European study. Curr Med Res Opin. 2005;21(11):1829–36.
4. van der Donk J, Passchier J, Dutree-Meulenberg RO, Stolz E, Verhage F. Psychologic characteristics of men with alopecia androgenetica and their modification. Int J Dermatol. 1991;30(1):22–8.
5. Girman CJ, Rhodes T, Lilly FR, Guo SS, Siervogel RM, Patrick DL, et al. Effects of self-perceived hair loss in a community sample of men. Dermatology. 1998;197(3):223–9.
6. Price VH. Androgenetic alopecia in adolescents. Cutis. 2003;71(2):115–21.
7. Wells PA, Willmoth T, Russell RJ. Does fortune favour the bald? Psychological correlates of hair loss in males. Br J Psychol. 1995;86(Pt 3):337–44.
8. Cash TF. The psychology of hair loss and its implications for patient care. Clin Dermatol. 2001;19(2):161–6.

9. Abt NB, Quatela O, Heiser A, Jowett N, Tessler O, Lee LN. Association of hair loss with health utility measurements before and after hair transplant surgery in men and women. JAMA Facial Plast Surg. 2018;20(6):495–500.
10. Rousso DE, Kim SW. A review of medical and surgical treatment options for androgenetic alopecia. JAMA Facial Plast Surg. 2014;16(6):444–50.
11. Bater KL, Ishii M, Joseph A, Su P, Nellis J, Ishii LE. Perception of hair transplant for androgenetic alopecia. JAMA Facial Plast Surg. 2016;18(6):413–8.
12. Konior RJ, Simmons C. Patient selection, candidacy, and treatment planning for hair restoration surgery. Facial Plast Surg Clin North Am. 2013;21(3):343–50.
13. Rebora A. Telogen effluvium: a comprehensive review. Clin Cosmet Investig Dermatol. 2019;12:583–90.
14. Lawenda BD, Gagne HM, Gierga DP, Niemierko A, Wong WM, Tarbell NJ, et al. Permanent alopecia after cranial irradiation: dose-response relationship. Int J Radiat Oncol Biol Phys. 2004;60(3):879–87.
15. Lee JA, Levy DA, Patel KG, Brennan E, Oyer SL. Hair transplantation in frontal fibrosing alopecia and lichen planopilaris: A systematic review. Laryngoscope. 2020;10.1002/lary.28551. https://doi:10.1002/lary.28551. PMID: 32045028.
16. Grant JE. Trichotillomania (hair pulling disorder). Indian J Psychiatry. 2019;61(Suppl 1):S136–S9.
17. Henkel ED, Jaquez SD, Diaz LZ. Pediatric trichotillomania: review of management. Pediatr Dermatol. 2019;36(6):803–7.

Designing the Hairline

Sahar Nadimi

Introduction

Creating a natural hairline is vital to a successful hair transplant. Modern hair trans-plantation techniques favor the exclusive use of follicular unit (FU) grafts to achieve recipient-site density and refinement. A better understanding of the visual character-istics that make up a normal hairline has also led to significant advances in hairline design [1–8].

Natural Characteristics of the Hairline

A natural frontal hairline is convex, with the central portion positioned slightly infe-rior to the frontotemporal triangle region. The lowest point of the midfrontal hair-line, the *trichion,* frames the superior face. Aesthetically, the youthful face is proportionately divided into vertical thirds with approximately equal distances observed between (1) the trichion and the glabella, (2) the glabella and the subna-sale, and (3) the subnasale and the mentum. In patients with more advanced hair loss, the newly created hairline is usually placed somewhat higher for a more aes-thetically acceptable, age-appropriate appearance. Depending on the degree of tem-poral recession and extent of balding, the lowest point of the hairline is generally placed approximately 7–10 cm superior to the glabella. Higher hairlines are gener-ally preferred for those with advanced hair-loss patterns and limited donor reserves [1, 2].

S. Nadimi (✉)
Department of Otolaryngology-Head and Neck Surgery,
Loyola University Medical Center, Maywood, IL, USA

Private Practice in Oakbrook Terrace, Maywood, IL, USA

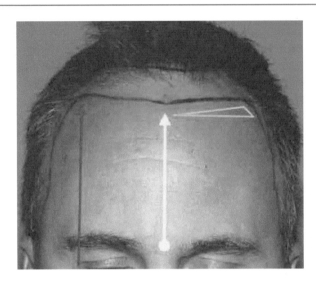

Fig. 5.1 Male hairline design. A natural male frontal hairline is convex, and the central portion is positioned slightly inferior to the lateral portion. The upper third of an aesthetically pleasing face extends from the glabella (*yellow dot*) to the trichion (*yellow arrow*). The central hairline is usually placed approximately 7–10 cm superior to the glabella. A mature male hairline usually demonstrates a distinct triangular region bilaterally at the junction of the frontal and the temporal hairlines (*blue triangle*). This triangle is formed by recession of the frontal hairline superiorly and the temporal hairline posteriorly. The apex of the frontotemporal triangle marks the lateral aspect of a natural frontal hairline and is usually located on a vertical line drawn upward from the lateral canthus of the eye (*red arrow*)

The mature male hairline usually demonstrates a distinct triangular region bilaterally at the junction of the frontal and the temporal hair. These frontotemporal triangles are formed by recession of the frontal hairline superiorly and the temporal hairline posteriorly. The ultimate goal of surgical hairline restoration is to recreate natural frontotemporal triangles, where the transplanted frontal hairline blends at its lateral edge with the naturally receding temporal fringe [2]. The apex of the frontotemporal triangle marks the lateral aspect of a natural hairline. Regardless of the extent of hairline recession, the apex is designed to fall on a vertical line drawn upward from the lateral canthus of the eye (Fig. 5.1). Because the temporal hairline intersects the lateral extent of the frontal hairline, advanced temporal recessions usually require a more posterior frontal hairline.

In certain ethnic groups (black, Middle Eastern, Asian, and Hispanic), it is more common to see broader, flatter hairlines with less recession [3]. In these patients, if the donor/recipient ratio is favorable, a more aggressively filled frontotemporal angle may be acceptable. However, even if a flatter hairline is more common in certain ethnic groups, some temporal recession still needs to be created if the donor/recipient ratio is unfavorable. With women, the frontotemporal angle is more medial, rounded, and filled in (Fig. 5.2).

Cowlicks can be a significant challenge when creating hairlines. If a patient has a residual cowlick that is very thin, it is reasonable to ignore it. However, if a

Fig. 5.2 Unlike the male hairline, the female hairline is characterized by a more medial, rounded, and filled in FTA

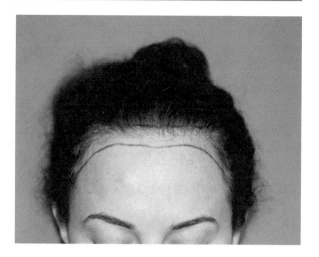

cowlick is strong, one may use the existing hairs as a road map to follow its direction. A cowlick can be re-created by starting at its periphery, where the direction of hair is obvious, and slowly work inward toward the point of swirl [3].

In general, the younger the patient, the more severe the hair loss, and the poorer the donor supply, the more conservative the hairline should be. It is important to explain to the patient that the donor area has a finite number of grafts and that we do not have an unlimited donor supply. If there is any concern, it is better to be conservative and create a higher hairline [1].

Although it is common for patients to have asymmetric hairline thinning, it is important to design a symmetric neohairline. Examining the hairline in a mirror or through a camera lens will often reveal asymmetry.

Components of the Hairline

The frontal hairline is an area that posteriorly extends approximately 2–3 cm, and consists of three zones: the anterior portion or transition zone (TZ), the posterior portion or defined zone (DZ), and an oval-shaped area in the center of the defined zone called the frontal tuft (FT) [2, 3] (Fig. 5.3).

The TZ consists of the first 1 cm of the hairline. One-hair grafts should be exclusively used in the anterior portion of the TZ with a shift toward two-hair grafts in the posterior portion. This helps to ensure a natural, softer look. Close examination of the hairline reveals small, intermittent clusters of hairs along its anterior border. These clusters vary in shape and depth but often resemble ill-defined triangles of various sizes. This form of irregularity, referred to as *microirregularity*, helps to prevent the creation of a straight or solid-appearing hairline (Fig. 5.4) [3, 9–11].

The DZ lies directly behind the TZ. The hairline should develop a higher degree of definition and density as larger follicular units are seen in this region. Increasing density in the DZ is an effective way to make the hairline appear thicker.

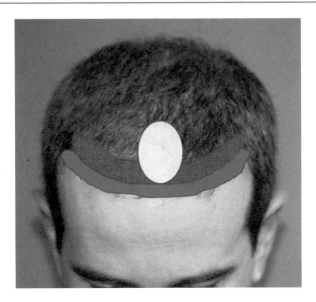

Fig. 5.3 The frontal hairline is an area that posteriorly extends approximately 2–3 cm, which consists of three zones: the anterior portion or transition zone (TZ) as seen in blue, the posterior portion or defined zone (DZ) as seen in red, and an oval-shaped area in the center of the defined zone called the frontal tuft (FT) as seen in yellow. The TZ consists of the first 1 cm of the hairline. One-hair grafts should be exclusively used in the anterior portion of the TZ. Posterior to this hairline transition zone, two-, three-, and four-hair FUs are used to provide density throughout the restoration area. The frontal tuft area contains a greater concentration of three-hair grafts

Fig. 5.4 The anterior hairline should be designed with small, intermittent clusters of hairs along its border (*white arrow*). These clusters vary in shape and depth but often resemble ill-defined triangles of various sizes. This form of irregularity is referred to as *microirregularity*. Microirregularity helps prevent the creation of a straight or solid-appearing hairline

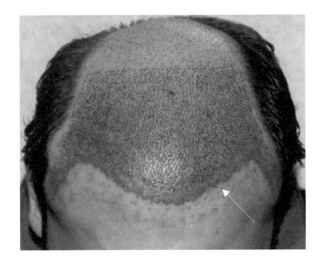

Within the central portion of the DZ lies the frontal tuft, a small but aesthetically significant oval-shaped area. The density in this area should be higher than the rest of the DZ. High-density grafting in the frontal tuft helps to create an overall appearance of fullness. For patients with advanced hair loss patterns, the frontal tuft is a key zone for graft placement.

Proper Angle and Direction

Most alopecic areas can be filled with dense-appearing hair in a single session, if the patient has an adequate donor supply. The original hair direction and exit angle must be followed carefully when creating recipient openings in order to maintain a natural hair growth pattern and to prevent transection of preexisting native hair [3].

Angle and direction are distinct entities. Angle refers to the degree of elevation that hair has as it exits the scalp. Direction refers to the way hair points (right or left) when leaving the scalp. It is important to pay attention to changes in both angle and direction as one transplants different parts of the hairline. Often there are residual miniaturized hairs that act as a road map for the physician to follow. Hair along the frontal hairline is usually directed anteriorly and exits the skin centrally at a 15- to 20-degree angle and laterally at a 10- to 15-degree angle (Fig. 5.5). Frontal hair direction reorients inferiorly toward the ear as the lateral hairline transitions into the temple region. This change requires grafts in the anterior temporal area to be placed with an inferior direction and a relatively flat 5- to 10-degree angle. Midscalp grafts are placed in a forward direction with a 30- to 45-degree exit angle to match the normal orientation of hair of this area [1, 3].

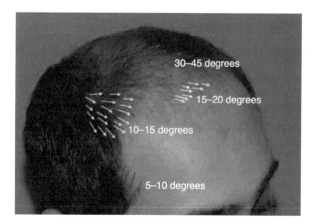

Fig. 5.5 Recipient-site incisions are made to control hair direction and angle. Hair in the central scalp is most commonly directed forward, with an exit angle of 30–45 degrees in the midscalp (*red arrows*) and 15–20 degrees at the hairline (*white arrows*). Hair direction begins to turn inferiorly toward the lateral aspect of the hairline and lays flatter, with an exit angle of 10–15 degrees in the frontotemporal region (*yellow arrows*). Anterior temporal hair is directed inferiorly and lays very flat at 5–10 degrees (*blue arrows*)

Selective Distribution of Grafts

Selective distribution of grafts is an important feature of a hair transplant to help recreate the density gradient found in normal hairlines. FUs are naturally occurring groups of one to four terminal hairs in which all of the support structures—including sebaceous glands, subcutaneous fat, and a circumferential band of perifollicular collagen—remain intact (Fig. 5.6). As previously discussed, the anterior frontal hairline (the TZ) is recreated exclusively with single-hair FUs to establish a natural "feathering" transition zone between the forehead and the higher density central scalp [2, 3]. Posterior to this hairline transition zone, two-, three-, and four-hair FUs are used to provide density throughout the restoration area. The frontal tuft area contains a greater concentration of three-hair grafts. A single-hair transition zone should also be created posteriorly if grafting stops short of a balding vertex. A higher density can be used in the part to compensate for the visually apparent density reduction that accompanies diverging hair along a part line. Recession of the temple points contributes a great deal to the appearance of baldness by making the forehead look larger. The angle of hair in the temple point should be flat or as close to zero as possible. The direction of hair points downward and posterior toward the ear. It is important to use single hair follicular units for the temporal points.

The recipient site is prepared for graft placement by making slits using flat-edge blades or needles. The slits typically measure 0.6–1.2 mm depending on the graft size. The depth of the incision is made to precisely accommodate the graft length, and grafts are spaced throughout the recipient site to ensure a balanced density

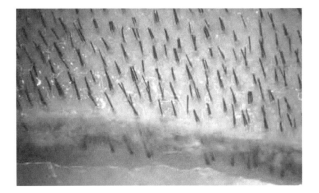

Fig. 5.6 Hair grows on the scalp in follicular units, which appear as discrete bundles that generally contain one to four hairs each. The success of follicular unit grafting depends in the meticulous isolation of these units under high-power magnification

Fig. 5.7 Recipient-site graft distribution. Grafts are evenly spaced to provide balanced coverage. Single-hair grafts are favored at the hairline for refinement, and two- to four-hair grafts are used further back to produce density. (**a**) A total of 1917 grafts were used to create a very natural and dense hairline in this female patient. (**b**) A total of 3058 grafts were transplanted in the front and midscalp to create a very natural and relatively dense appearance in this male patient

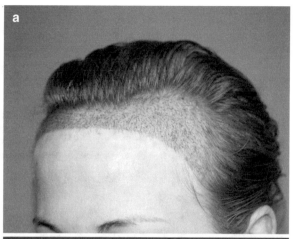

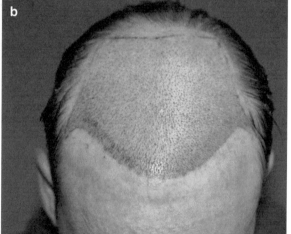

distribution (Fig. 5.7). Incisions are made, taking care to preserve an intact, circumferential bridge of skin between adjacent openings to ensure optimal circulatory conditions around each graft.

Microforceps are used to place grafts into the individual recipient slits, giving attention to ensure proper depth and rotational relationships. Grafts must be kept moist at all times and are placed atraumatically by grasping the surrounding fat in order to preserve follicular viability and optimize graft yield.

The final result following the strategic planning and placement of individual FUs is a predictably natural look (Figs. 5.8, 5.9, and 5.10).

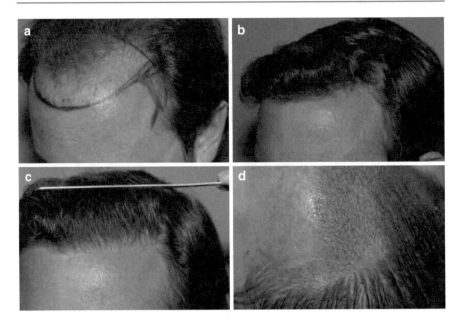

Fig. 5.8 Follicular unit hairline restoration. A total of 3252 grafts were used to create a very natural and relatively dense appearance in this class IV balding pattern. (**a**) Preoperative view. (**b**) Postoperative view. (**c**) Postoperative view with hair combed back. (**d**) Immediate postoperative graft distribution shows proper direction and a natural appearance

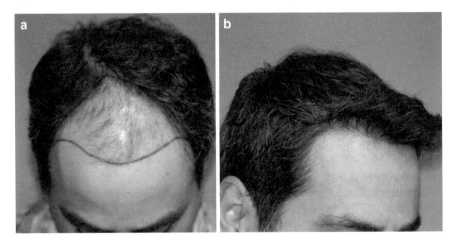

Fig. 5.9 Follicular unit hairline restoration. A total of 2200 grafts were used to create a very natural and relatively dense hairline and midscalp. (**a**) Preoperative view. (**b**) Postoperative view. (**c**) Postoperative view with hair combed back. (**d**) Immediate postoperative graft distribution shows proper direction and a natural appearance

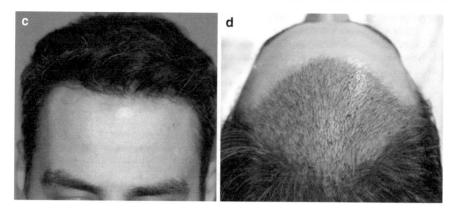

Fig. 5.9 (continued)

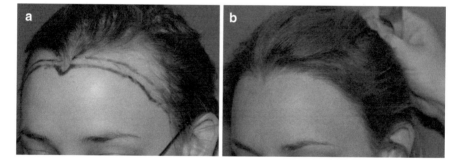

Fig. 5.10 Follicular unit hairline restoration. A total of 1800 grafts were used to create a very natural and relatively dense hairline. (**a**) Preoperative view. (**b**) Postoperative view

Conclusion

A better understanding and recognition of the visual characteristics that make up a normal hairline has led to significant advances in hairline design. Modern hair transplantation techniques favor the exclusive use of follicular unit (FU) grafts to achieve recipient-site density, refinement, and a predictably natural look. With proper planning and precise execution of the plan, a natural hairline can be achieved for patients.

References

1. Konior RJ, Nadimi S. Hair restoration. In: Flint PW, editor. Cummings otolaryngology: head & neck surgery. 7th ed. Philadelphia: Elsevier; In press. Chapter 22.
2. Shapiro R. Creating a natural hairline in one session using a systematic approach and modern principles of hairline design. Int J Cosmet Surg Aesthet Dermatol. 2001;3(2):89–99.

3. Shapiro R, Shapiro P. Hairline design and frontal hairline restoration. Facial Plast Surg Clin North Am. 2013;21:351–62.
4. Unger W. Hairline zone. In: Unger W, Shapiro R, editors. Hair transplantation. 5th ed. New York: Informa; 2011. p. 133–40. Chapter 6A.
5. Shapiro R. How to use follicular unit transplantation in the hairline and other appropriate areas. In: Unger WP, Shapiro R, editors. Hair transplantation. 4th ed. New York: Marcel Dekker; 2004. p. 454–69.
6. Stough D, Khan S. Determination of hairline placement. In: Stough D, Haber R, editors. Hair replacement: surgical and medical: Mosby-Year Book. St. Louis: Mosby; 1996. p. 425–9.
7. Rose PT, Parsley WM. The science of hairline design. In: Haber RS, Stough DB, editors. Procedures in cosmetic dermatology. Hair transplantation. Philadelphia: Elsevier Saunders; 2006. p. 55–72.
8. Lam S. Hairline design. In: Hair transplant 360. Philadelphia: Jay-pee Brothers Medical Pub; 2011. Ch 50.
9. McAndrews P. Hairlines based on natural patterns of hair loss. In: Unger W, Shapiro R, editors. Hair transplantation. 5th ed. New York: Informa; 2011. p. 152–62. Chapter 6B1.
10. Parsley WM. Natural hair patterns. Facial Plast Surg Clin North Am. 2004;12:167–80.
11. Shapiro R. Principles and techniques used to create a natural hairline in surgical hair restoration. Facial Plast Surg Clin North Am. 2004;12:201–17.

Follicular Unit Transplant Technique

6

Sarina K. Mueller, Linda N. Lee, and Samuel L. Oyer

Follicular Unit Transplant

Key Principles

- Definition of a follicular unit: Naturally occurring group of 1–4 hairs surrounded by sebaceous glands, nerves, erector pili muscle, and supporting fat and stroma.
- Follicular unit transplant (FUT or strip harvest) and follicular unit extraction (FUE) techniques differ primarily in how the donor hair is *harvested*. It is important for the patient to understand that *placement of the hair into the recipient sites* is performed the same way regardless of whether FUT or FUE transplant is chosen.
- In both FUT and FUE techniques, the transplanted hair is harvested from a safe donor area at the occiput that consists of permanent hair resistant to androgenetic hair loss.
- The FUT harvest results in a thin, linear scar that is usually well covered by the surrounding occipital hair if the hair is at least ½ inch long. Modern techniques including a trichophytic, meticulous, tension-free closure can help to minimize the appearance of the donor site scar by allowing remaining hair to grow through the scar for additional camouflage.

S. K. Mueller (✉)
Friedrich-Alexander-Universität Erlangen-Nürnberg (FAU), Department of Otolaryngology, Head and Neck Surgery, Erlangen, Germany
e-mail: sarina.mueller@uk-erlangen.de

L. N. Lee
Facial Plastic and Reconstructive Surgery, Assistant Professor, Harvard Medical School, Massachusetts Eye and Ear, Associate Chief of Plastic Surgery, Harvard Vanguard Medical Associates, Boston, MA, USA

S. L. Oyer
Facial Plastic & Reconstructive Surgery, University of Virginia, Charlottesville, VA, USA

© Springer Nature Switzerland AG 2020
L. N. Lee (ed.), *Hair Transplant Surgery and Platelet Rich Plasma*,
https://doi.org/10.1007/978-3-030-54648-9_6

- If subsequent FUT transplant is desired in the future, the excision can be designed to incorporate the original scar.
- If multiple FUT transplants are performed and there is limited scalp laxity, FUE transplant can be performed following or concurrent with FUT transplants (i.e., the initial choice of FUT or FUE does not obligate the patient to undergo the same technique in procedures).

History of FUT Hair Transplantation

Hair loss is a common and often progressive condition that affects patients of all ages, races, and genders. For some patients, hair loss may be caused by natural aging along with a genetic and hormonal predisposition, while in others it is a sign of an underlying medical condition. Despite the high prevalence and overall benign nature of hair loss, many patients suffer from significant negative psychosocial effects such as reduced self-esteem and self-confidence [1] along with a reduced perception of attractiveness, likeability, and overall success by others [2, 3]. These factors have spurred an intense social interest in camouflaging or combatting hair loss for centuries and multiple medical and surgical treatments have been devised with varying success. Arguably, the first hair transplant procedure was reported by Hodara [4] in 1897, and eyebrow and eyelash transplant techniques were first described in Japan in the 1930s [5]. The modern era of hair transplantation began in the late 1950s in New York, when N. Orentreich [6] identified the concept of donor dominance and used free donor occipital grafts to areas of hair loss in patients with male pattern baldness. This concept remains the fundamental foundation for hair transplant success to this day and laid the groundwork for hair follicle harvesting, whether by strip technique (follicular unit transplant: FUT) or by follicular unit extraction (FUE).

Initial hair grafts consisted of 4 mm punch biopsies each containing 15–20 hairs which allowed for permanent hair survival and growth when transplanted to the areas of hair loss in the anterior scalp, but produced an un-natural "doll's head" appearance. Further refinements in the 1980s consisted of dividing these grafts into smaller and smaller segments including minigrafts (5–10 hairs) and micrografts (1–4 hairs). Headington [7] described the concept of the follicular unit in 1984 as a natural grouping of 1–4 hairs along with associated sebaceous glands, neurovascular plexus, erector pili muscle, and fine villous hairs. This anatomical description defined safe borders between follicular units to allow for even smaller dissection of viable grafts into individual follicular units for transplant. Strip harvest was popularized over punch graft excision, and in 1994, Limmer first described the use of the stereomicroscope to dissect a single donor strip into small micrografts [8], thus the modern era of FUT was born. This same year Walter Unger [9] defined the parameters of the "Safe Donor Zone" from which the most permanent hair follicles could be extracted for hair transplantation and further refinements were made in hairline design and recipient site creation to improve the natural appearance of hair transplant results. Improved efficiency of harvesting and dissecting allowed surgeons such as Rassmann to transplant thousands of "micrografts" in a single session [10].

Over the years and numerous iterations, FUT has reliably produced a very safe, outpatient method of hair replacement surgery effective for both male and female pattern alopecia. Modern FUT technique and meticulous attention to detail can now provide very natural appearing results, especially with recent advances such as single hair follicular unit hairline reconstruction, irregularization of the hairline, improved understanding of angles and density for transplantation of the grafts, and trichophytic donor site closure techniques [11]. Recent studies of public perception after hair transplant surgery demonstrate that patients after transplant appear younger, more attractive, more successful, and approachable with higher health utility scores [12, 13].

Goals/Realistic Expectations

The goal of every transplant is to achieve a natural appearing result with which the patient can age gracefully. In deciding between FUT and FUE techniques, a detailed discussion should be undertaken with the patient regarding preferred hairstyles, personal and family history of hair loss, and most importantly, the possible need for additional transplants as hair loss progresses in the future. All hair transplant results should ideally mimic a *naturally occurring* hair loss pattern along the Norwood classification scheme for men and Ludwig classification for women. Patients who are at the severe ends of these scales cannot be completely restored to a full head of hair due to constraints between supply and demand (e.g., a patient who is Norwood stage VI cannot be restored to a Norwood stage II pattern of hair loss). A patient's treatment goals may need to be tempered in light of the amount of donor hair available for transplant. Restoring a patient's hair pattern to something outside of the naturally occurring patterns will *always* appear unnatural regardless of the skill and precision of the transplant itself.

Patients must understand that while the transplanted hair will be permanent, loss of the native surrounding hair may still progress. Here, the physician should emphasize the benefit of continued medical management of hair loss covered in *Chap. 3* of this textbook which will support the surrounding hairs and help limit future loss. While it is never possible to predict exactly the future extent of a hair loss for an individual, the patient's age and a detailed family history of hair loss should be considered and a "worse-case scenario" discussed with each patient. This will help guide the patient–physician discussion toward goals of hair transplant, prioritize areas for treatment, and determine the extent of reconstruction to undertake at the onset along with the possible need for future transplants. For example, if the temples or anterior hairline are aggressively transplanted in a young patient with a profound family history of hair loss, and then the central forelock and midscalp hair is lost in the future, the patient will have a very unnatural appearing result and look worse than if no transplant was undertaken. In this case, the patient would be committing themselves to additional transplants in the future to camouflage the newly balding areas. Alternatively, a middle-aged man with a Norwood V pattern of hair loss may wish to restore his frontal hairline and his crown. Given the large number of grafts needed to restore the crown, he may be better served by transplanting the hairline and midscalp to achieve a Norwood III-vertex pattern of hair loss to frame his face from the frontal view, with fewer if any grafts devoted to less commonly viewed crown. Patients should not undergo and initial transplant unless they understand this possibility of needing a subsequent transplant in the future. Based upon the patient's treatment goals and commitment to continued medical management after transplant, it would be far wiser to decline to operate on a patient with unrealistic goals than to perform a transplant which gives an unnatural look or does not hold up to future hair loss.

Indications and Contraindications for FUT

Indications

FUT involves excising a strip of scalp with direct surgical closure. This creates a linear scar along the occipital scalp which is generally well hidden if the occipital hair is worn long enough. Only the strip of scalp that is being removed requires clipping at the time of surgery, so the surrounding hair will cover the incision even with sutures in place immediately after surgery. FUE, in contrast, often requires closely clipping hair for a larger portion of the back of the scalp and takes individual grafts from a broader scalp area with small, circular punches which heal secondarily. Contrary to marketing claims, FUE is not "scar-less surgery," but the scars are instead small circular gaps in hair growth that are generally less visible than a linear scar for patients who wear their hair extremely short. Indications for FUT harvest include:

- Most women are excellent candidates for the FUT technique as hairstyles are often long enough to hide the scar and many women are opposed to clipping a large section of hair short enough for standard FUE harvest (see Fig. 6.1).
- Men with androgenic alopecia who wear their hair longer than a #3 guard haircut and who do not plan on shaving their heads in the future.
- Adequate donor hair density in the occipital scalp to meet transplant needs.
- Adequate scalp laxity to allow for direct closure. This is best assessed by manually pinching the scalp to determine mobility.

Contraindications

All patients should be considered on an individual basis, and risks and benefits assessed carefully. Historically, patients with scarring alopecias were considered contraindications for hair transplant, but recent small studies have shown benefit

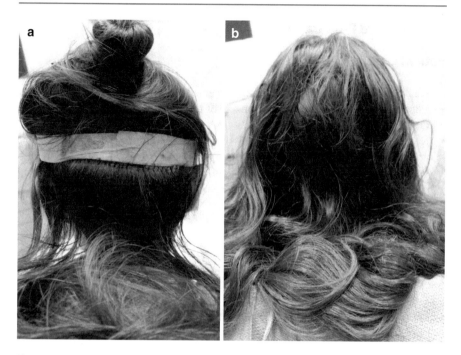

Fig. 6.1 (**a**) For this woman with long hair in the donor region, FUT was chosen over FUE because of time and cost-efficiency. FUT also did not require shaving of her donor site hair (**b**) Immediately after FUT harvest, with sutures in place, the incision is well-concealed

in some patients with stable disease [14]. As such, all contraindications are considered relative contraindications and should be discussed in detail together with the patient.

- Extremely short hairstyle or possible future desire to shave head (FUE preferred)
- Young age with unstable hair loss
- Any patient with unrealistic expectations
- Generalized thinning (including the donor site)
- History of keloid scars or poor scarring
- Inelastic scalp which would limit closure (FUE preferred)
- Smoking or history of scalp radiation
- History of bleeding disorders
- Active vitiligo or other disease of the skin
- History of Koebner phenomenon
- Scarring alopecias (may be considered in some quiescent cases, but expectations should be downgraded)
- Telogen effluvium (usually self-limited and hair transplant not needed)
- Alopecia areata (usually treated medically and hair transplant is rarely indicated)

Preoperative Preparation

Patient Comfort

- Hair transplant is a lengthy procedure and ensuring patient comfort is paramount.
- Local anesthetic blocks are the mainstay of analgesia during the procedure.
- Oral anxiolytics or for some, IV sedation, may improve patient comfort.
- No fasting is required and patients are encouraged to take breaks during the procedure.
- Patients are encouraged to use audio or video entertainment during portions of the procedure.

Equipment

Hair transplant is considered a clean, but not strictly sterile procedure. The following is a list of commonly used instruments for FUT harvest (Fig. 6.2):

- Paper tape to uphold the hair during the procedure; for women, additional hair clips might be needed.
- One permanent marker.
- Electric razor.
- Lidocaine with epinephrine (1:100,000) for anesthetic and vasoconstrictive effect.
- Blue towels for prepping and draping.
- Backhaus/penetrating towel clamp.
- Five mosquito clamps.
- Fine scissors.
- 10 blade scalpel.
- Needle driver.
- Single-toothed forceps.
- Cotton swabs.
- Gauze sponges.

Fig. 6.2 Surgical equipment for harvesting the strip, trichophytic closure and making the slit incisions for transplanting the follicular units

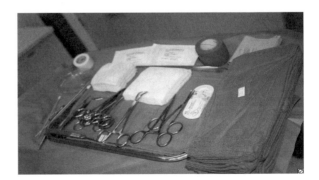

- 2 sutures of 4-0 Prolene (Prolene monofil blue FS 2S needle, 45 cm, nonabsorbable).
- 3-0 silks (if needed for ligation of small bleeding vessels).
- One petri dish with chilled storage solution.

Operative Technique

Designing the Donor Strip

Safe Donor Area   The donor hair can be harvested from the safe donor area (SDA) of the permanent hair which can be found postauricular in the occipital scalp (for further information, please see *Chap. 3: Hair Loss Physiology and Transplantation Principles*). The SDA is bordered anteriorly by a vertical line drawn from the external auditory canal and runs as a half-circle around the occiput. This region is more superiorly positioned in the temple and dips inferiorly in the occipital scalp. According to the safe donor zone suggested by Alt [15], the superior border of SDA in the temple can extend up to 6.5–7 cm above the intersection of the anterior helix skin and the temporal scalp hair. The superior border of the SDA in the occipital scalp is defined as the intersection of the midline of the occiput and a horizontal line that is drawn 2 cm superior to the junction of the anterior helix and the temporal scalp hair. It is recommended to preserve at least 2.5 cm of hair above the upper edge of donor zone to ensure enough hair remains to camouflage the donor scar. The inferior border of the SDA is determined by examination and family history, but it should stay above the external occipital protuberance in the occiput for ease of closure (Fig. 6.3).

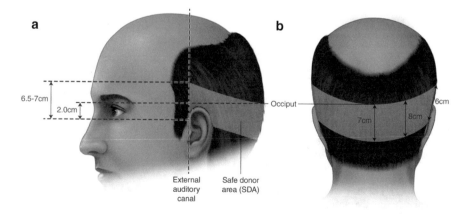

Fig. 6.3   Boundaries of the safe donor area (SDA) shown from lateral (**a**) and occipital (**b**) views

Width of the Donor Strip Design a strip of approximately 1 cm width within the SDA based on scalp laxity. If the scalp shows minimal laxity, or in case of a revision procedure, the strip width should be restricted to 0.8 cm. In a virgin scalp with excellent laxity, a strip width of 1.2 cm can be considered. Keep in mind that the area of greatest tension on closure occurs in the postauricular area over the bony mastoid.

Length of the Donor Strip The length of the donor strip incision is determined by the number of follicular unit grafts required for the hair restoration (for further information concerning the hairline design, see *Chap. 5*). Follicular unit density in the donor area can vary by location and between patients, so it is important to get a good estimate of donor density for each patient when determining the length of the strip needed. After the hair is trimmed, density can be determined most accurately by viewing the donor area through a magnified densitometer to count the number of follicular units (FU) per cm^2. This may be higher in the occiput and slightly lower in the temples, so it is useful to take several measurements across the entire donor area to get an accurate count. Generally, the donor scalp with have a density around 80 FU/cm^2 so a transplant requiring 2000 grafts with a 1 cm wide strip would require a strip length of 25 cm (25 cm × 1 cm × 80 FU/cm^2 = 2000 FU grafts). A 1.2 cm wide strip would only need to be 21 cm long to achieve the same number of grafts (21 cm × 1.2 cm × 80 FU/cm^2 = 2016 FU grafts).

Harvesting the Donor Strip

Preparation First, mark the incision with a ruler and a permanent marker. Never infiltrate any local anesthetic prior to marking, as this will change your dimensions. Then, use paper tape to secure the hair above the incision precisely. This step is important as it can prevent shaving the hair above the marked strip, which can after the procedure cover the sutures (Fig. 6.4). For women with long hair, additional clips or hair tape might be needed to keep hair out of the field.

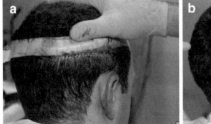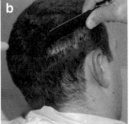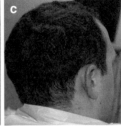

Fig. 6.4 (**a**) The hair superior to the strip is carefully taped upward prior to the harvest. Immediately after the closure of the donor site, the prolene sutures are visible. (**b**) After the tape is removed, the hair can be combed to strategically cover the sutures. (**c**) The sutures are not visible because they are covered by the remnant occipital hair

Using an electric trimmer, cut the hair in the donor strip to a length of about 5 mm. It may be helpful to extend the trimmed area a few millimeter past the marked incisions to ensure that no hair is trapped into the wound during closure. A ring block is then performed inferior to the marked strip with lidocaine with epinephrine (1:100,000) for anesthetic and vasoconstrictive effect (for further information, see *Chap. 8*). Once the anesthetic has taken effect, dilute tumescence should be infiltrated into the dermal plane along the length of the donor strip to make the scalp taught. This helps limit bleeding during harvest, minimizes follicle transection by slightly spreading follicles apart, and decreases risk of injury to underlying neurovascular structures in the galeal level by lifting the subcutaneous tissue away from this plane.

Incision Wait for the full vasoconstrictive effect before using a blade to incise the donor strip. The authors prefer a 10 blade. Start at the inferior aspect of the incision to allow any blood to drip down without interfering with the surgical site and carefully bevel parallel to the hair follicles in order to prevent transection of the follicles. Go slowly and stop intermittently to reevaluate that no transection has occurred keeping in mind that the direction of follicles varies in different locations across the scalp; tighter angle close to the scalp in the temples and angled further away from the scalp in the occiput. The ideal depth of the incision should be immediately below the hair follicles in the subcutaneous layer. If an incision is performed too deep, excessive bleeding is more likely and the incision should not extend to the galeal layer. Next, the superior edge of the incision can be carried out in a similar fashion and the two incisions tapered to meet at each end, again observing follicle angle the entire time to minimize transection. After a complete incision, the lateral corner should be grasped with a toothed forcep or a penetrating towel clamp to place the strip on some tension. With the help of the tension from the nondominant hand pulling on the strip, the 10 blade or blunt-tipped scissors can be used to cut preserving ~1 mm of fat deep to the follicle root and remove the strip in a sharp fashion (see Fig. 6.5).

Fig. 6.5 Elevating the strip in the subcutaneous plane immediately deep to the follicles. Note the hemostasis achieved through local injection and tumescence

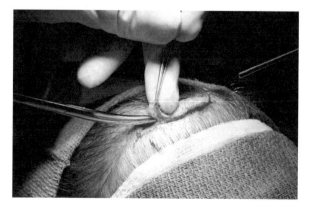

Graft Preparation

Immediately after removing the strip (Fig. 6.6), this is passed off in the cooled stor-age solution to the hair technicians for further microscopic dissection. In cases where the follicular unit density varies across the length of the strip or where exact follicular unit count is critical, the surgeon can consider sectioning a defined length of the strip (1–2 cm) and passing this off for graft dissection and counting while the remainder of the strip is being harvested. This can allow a more accurate estimate of grafts available in the donor strip including the relative proportion of grafts contain-ing 1, 2, 3, or 4 hairs. If the follicular unit yield determined by initial strip dissection varies from the estimates based on density, the surgeon can adjust the strip length or width slightly as needed to obtain the desired number of grafts.

Working under a binocular stereomicroscope, the surgical hair technicians ini-tially sliver the strip into single file rows of hair follicles which are subsequently dissected into individual follicular units (see Fig. 6.7). Each graft is carefully trimmed to ensure uniform sizing of the epithelial portion and the small amount of

Fig. 6.6 Sample donor strip after FUT harvest

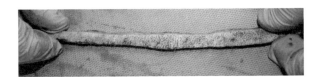

Fig. 6.7 Hair technician performing slivering and dissection of the harvested strip into follicular unit grafts using the stereomicroscope

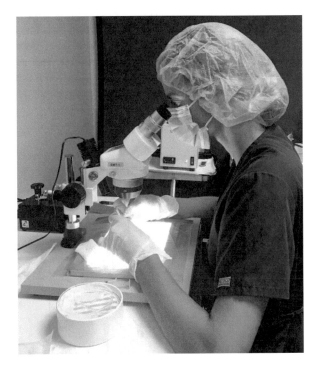

fat left around the hair bulb, and the grafts are sorted based on the number of hairs each graft contains (Fig. 6.8). During microdissection, it is critical to keep the grafts chilled and moist in an appropriate storage solution to maximize graft survival. Grafts prepared following FUT harvest tend to be a little thicker with more fatty tissue surrounding the hair shaft and bulb than grafts obtained by FUE which have very little fat beneath the hair bulb. This may allow for slightly improved graft survival among FUT grafts relative to FUE and may also impact the size of the recipient sites needed for each type of graft. Details of graft slivering and dissection are beyond the scope of this textbook, but meticulous attention to detail in this step is critical for graft survival and transplant success.

Fig. 6.8 (**a**) Close-up view of the FUT strip after harvest – beveling of the incision is important to minimize transection of any follicles, especially along the edges of the strip. (**b**) Individual follicular units after slivering and dissecting of the grafts. This is performed manually under microscopic assistance on the back table by experienced hair technicians

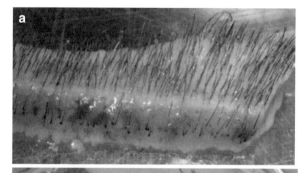

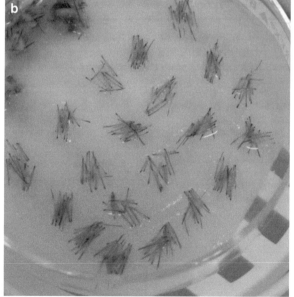

Hemostasis

Mosquito clamps (snaps) should be used to clamp any bleeding areas that do not stop with pressure alone (Fig. 6.9). Any significant bleeding vessels may be tied off with a 3-0 silk, but most commonly light diffuse bleeding will stop with temporary pressure from the clamp. Consider bipolar coagulation judiciously if needed, but utmost care should be taken to avoid cauterizing near any follicles if possible. Light bleeding from the skin edges will typically stop when the incision is closed with sutures.

Trichophytic Closure

Attention to detail during wound closure is just as critical as during strip harvest to avoid undermining an excellent transplant outcome with a visible or poorly healed scar. Due to the unnatural linearity of the scar after strip incision using FUT, the resulting scar might be visible in patients with a short haircut particularly if there is reduced hair growth in the scar itself. The trichophytic closure technique aims to limit the visibility of the final scar by encouraging hair growth through the scar. The principle of the trichophytic closure has previously been described in other aesthetic and reconstructive surgeries of the face and the scalp, but the term was first coined by Mayer and Flemming [16] in 1992. Kridel et al. utilized the technique which they called "hair camouflage incision" to hide temporal facelift scars [17]. The trichophytic closure technique was first described almost simultaneously by Marzola, Rose, and Frechet for donor area management after hair transplants [18–21]. Many hair transplant surgeons routinely utilize this technique and consider it the gold standard closure technique after FUT strip excision.

Fig. 6.9 After the harvest, mosquito clamps and 3-0 silk ties are used for hemostasis. Bipolar cauterization can be used judiciously, but monopolar cautery should be avoided if possible

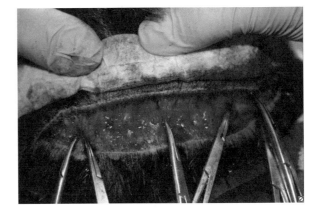

Key Principles

- The upper portion of follicles and epithelium of one wound edge is intentionally transected with a beveled cut.
- The intact skin edge is sutured to the de-epithelialized edge with slight overlap to allow the cutaneous scar and follicles to be slightly offset.
- Single layer closure with permanent running suture placed at the midpoint of the hair shaft is usually sufficient.
- A few months postoperatively, the hair regrows through the scar ensuring minimal visibility of the scar.

Indications

- Patients after FUT excision with adequate scalp laxity and good donor density who wish to maximally camouflage the donor scar.

Contraindications/Limitations

- A tight scalp with limited laxity of the skin, or projected need for multiple transplants.
- Previous scarring or procedures which make closure more difficult.
- Fine caliber or poor density of hair in safe donor area.
- Projected need for maximal use of donor hair in a patient who intends to always keep their occipital hair long. The trichophytic closure potentially sacrifices a row of hair follicles to limit scar visibility. In some patients who desire a longer hairstyle and need the maximum amount of grafts, the trichophytic closure may be omitted in favor of maximizing graft yield.

Technique

After strip excision, the resulting wound consists of an upper and lower skin edge with a roughly uniform bevel parallel to the remaining row of hair follicles on either side. Wound tension should be evaluated manually as the upper and lower skin edges are temporarily brought together with penetrating towel clamps. If the edges meet easily with minimal tension, the trichophytic closure technique can be utilized, but if there is any significant tension on the skin edges, the surgeon should consider forgoing trichophytic closure in favor or direct linear closure. Donor sites that are closed under tension create a scenario prime for vascular compromise of the skin edges and wound dehiscence which heals with a much more unsightly scar than direct non-trichophytic closure creates, not to mention a much less satisfied patient regardless of the recipient site success. If trichophytic closure is selected, an angled incision roughly 1 mm deep is made to de-epithelialize the skin and intentionally transect the upper portion of hair follicles along one of the skin edges over the complete length of the flap. Specialized instruments like the Puig-Barusco ledge spacer knife that exposes only 1–1.5 mm of the scalpel tip can be used to create this cut, but sharp tenotomy scissors or a 15-blade can be easily used as well. After the transection, the flap should appear from a lateral view as if you have excised a small

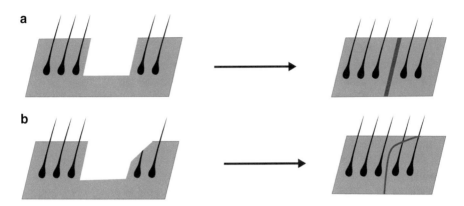

Fig. 6.10 (a) Wound bed after strip harvest without trichophytic closure results in linear scar with some space between neighboring rows of follicles. (b) Wound bed after trichophytic closure with excision of epithelium and partial transection of hair follicles on the inferior skin flap. The epithelium of the superior skin flap is overlapped over the transected follicle of the inferior edge allowing the hair to regrow through the scar and minimize scar visibility

1 mm wide × 0.5–1 mm deep edge over the complete length of the strip (see Fig. 6.10). Technically, this procedure can be performed for the inferior or the superior flap, however, the inferior flap is favored for transection due to the natural overhang of the superior skin flap and hair direction of the occipital hair which drapes over the exposed beveled inferior flap [22]. By de-epithelializing the flap, the underlying follicles are also superficially transected. The optimal depth of the transection takes the epidermis and a small part of the papillary dermis [23]. Deeper excision might damage the follicles which can result in poor or no regrowth of hair.

The wound is closely examined and any stray hair remnants are carefully removed, then the inferior and the superior flaps are sutured together. The authors prefer single layer closure with a 4-0 prolene suture (Prolene monofil blue FS 2S needle, 45 cm). Undermining of the skin edges prior to closure should be avoided as much as possible to preserve unscarred hair follicles that can be used for future hair transplants if needed. Consideration should be given to allowing the towel clamps to remain in place for several minutes to achieve slight mechanical creep or injecting hyaluronidase into both edges of the defect if there is tension perceived during closure. If undermining is performed, take care to undermine deep to the level of the follicular bulb to avoid injury to the follicles, and the galeal layer should not be disrupted [23]. The de-epithelialized edge should be slightly overlapped by the opposite flap. *When closing, the depth of the needle should remain superficial to the bulb of the follicle around mid-shaft to avoid damage and prevent hair loss.* Care should also be taken to place sutures between the hairs as much as possible to minimize trauma to the follicles. The authors prefer using segments of running suture, rather than a single running suture.

Following closure, the wound should be cleaned with a spray bottle of hydrogen peroxide and saline mixed 50:50. Remove the tape and comb the hair over the incision. Many patients appreciate seeing the donor site after closure, to reassure them that the incision is not visible. This can be done by giving the patient a mirror while holding a second mirror behind the head. This may help allay any worries the patient has about the visibility of the scar for the remainder of the case.

Graft Placement

The primary difference between FUT and FUE techniques centers around how the donor hair is harvested. Once the follicles are harvested and isolated into individual follicular unit grafts, placing them into the desired area is performed in the same manner whether FUT or FUE was used for graft harvest. The surgeon should mark the designed hairline or recipient area with a permanent marker. This marking should be shown to the patient and modified as needed to ensure that both patient and surgeon agree. Nerve blocks can be performed at this time. Local injection of short and long-acting anesthetic, as well as tumescence is performed to aid with hemostasis. (See *Chap. 8* for a description of the injection techniques). While awaiting adequate time for vasoconstriction and anesthesia, blades are prepared according to the individual patient's hair characteristics. Multiple blade and needle options exist for customizing the incision depth and width of each follicular unit graft. These include solid or hollow, round, or slit-shaped instruments. Regardless of the specific blades or needles chosen for the case, attention should be given to matching the natural width and length of the patient's hair follicle for each area that is to be transplanted. For example, when creating a hairline, the surgeon may choose to use a finer, smaller blade for the first few rows of single hair follicular units, and posterior to that may use a slightly wider blade to place 2–3 hair follicular units, with a larger size yet for the midscalp and crown for 3–4 hair follicular units to maximize density. All the individual incisions are made by the surgeon under loupe magnification. For the most natural appearance, intentional irregularization is performed for recipient sites in the anterior hairline, and incisions are made in a staggered, interlocking fashion to avoid creating a linear row of hairs [24]. Single follicular units should be placed on the anterior hairline to avoid a "pluggy" doll-like appearance and soften the hairline [25]. The goal is to trick the eye into thinking the reconstructed hairline is naturally occurring. If there are surrounding existing hairs in the recipient region, care is taken to parallel the direction of these hairs and avoid transecting viable follicles. If there are no surrounding hairs, it is critical to align the recipient sites with the correct angle and inclination of natural hairs at that location in the scalp. These angles vary considerably by the location on the scalp, and a natural flow of hair angle and inclination is critical to produce a natural appearance [26]. It is also important for the surgeon to keep track of the number of recipient sites created with each size of blade to ensure that this matches the number of grafts that are prepared by the hair technicians. Once all recipient sites are created by the surgeon, the grafts can then be placed individually by the hair technicians (Fig. 6.11).

Fig. 6.11 The recipient sites have all been made, and the hair technicians now begin placing each graft into the sites

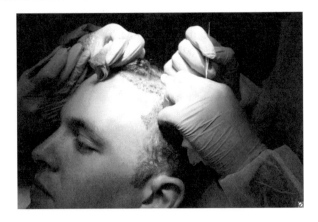

Graft placement represents another critical step in the process which much be completed quickly and carefully keeping the grafts moist and minimizing trauma to the grafts while following the angled direction of the sites created by the surgeon. This is a good opportunity for final quality control by all the team members to ensure the grafts are seating into the sites appropriately. The epithelial portion of the graft should rest ~1 mm higher than the surrounding scalp skin and the direction of the hair shaft should match the desired direction of the recipient site. The insertion of the follicular units in the preformed sites preserves the elasticity of the scalp and holds the fragile grafts in place. After surgery, the tight fit facilitates wound healing and helps to ensure that the grafts will get enough oxygen and nutrients from the surrounding tissue to maximize their survival [27].

Postoperative Care

- No dressings or bandages are needed.
- The patient should keep the grafts moist by spraying grafts with saline or liposomal ATP solution every 1–2 hours for the first 48 hours.
- A light head covering or hat may be worn if desired and should not fit tightly around the scalp.
- The patient is usually advised to sleep relatively upright or elevated for the next 3–5 days to avoid unwanted gravitational pull on the grafts, or unintentional rolling onto the recipient area.
- Swelling of the forehead is commonly seen in the first few days following the procedure and may be reduced with head elevation and ice to the forehead (not the grafts).
- Shampooing the hair is usually recommended twice a day, starting ~48 hours after the procedure, but this is done with a gentle technique.
- Donor site sutures are typically removed in 1–2 weeks.
- Cutting or coloring the hair can be resumed after 2 weeks.
- Most patients return to work after 1–2 weeks after the procedure.

- Counsel the patients that early results can be expected after 6–8 months.
- Full results can be expected after 1 year.
- In both FUT and FUE techniques, patients should be advised during the preoperative visit about the possibility of telogen effluvium (temporary loss of hair in the recipient scalp), which can occur in the first 3–4 months after surgery.

Complications

In general, a properly performed FUT with trichophytic closure is a safe technique with satisfying results for the patients. However, there is a low risk of complications which should be discussed with the patient:

- Excessive bleeding (more common if the plane of dissection is too deep)
- Persistent numbness from nerve injury
- Permanent damage of the follicular units and loss of hair density
- Visible, widened, or keloid scar
- Incision dehiscence/skin necrosis and resulting poor wound healing
- Donor or recipient site infection
- Poor growth of transplanted grafts
- Unnatural appearance of transplanted grafts despite good growth
- Incorrect hair angle or depth (i.e., pitting or prominence of the grafts)
- Milia or folliculitis at graft site (this common postoperative finding should be discussed with patients upfront and is easily managed with topical compresses or unroofing)
- Patient dissatisfaction

Tips and Pearls and Expert Suggestions

- If the full donor strip length is not needed, ask the patient which side they usually sleep on and harvest from the opposite side, since the donor site will be tender to lie on postoperatively. Patients can use an airplane neck pillow while sleeping to decrease the pressure placed on the donor incision. Pressure on the donor site is not medically contraindicated, but may be uncomfortable for the patient during sleep.
- If a second or third hair transplant is desired, place the superior part of the donor strip in the prior scar and design the new strip extending inferior from this point. Using this technique, assuming adequate scalp laxity, the scar will remain narrow and in the same place even after multiple procedures.
- If there is poor scalp laxity following initial FUT transplant, more donor follicles can be obtained using the FUE method during future transplants.
- Prior to closing the donor site, multiple penetrating towel clamps may be used to bring the two sides of the donor site closer and reduce tension using mechanical

creep. The towel clamps are removed sequentially as the incision is closed. Hyaluronidase can be injected into the wound edges for particularly tight scalps.

- While performing trichophytic closure, do not incise deeper than 1.5 mm as the bulge of the follicles lays about 2–4 mm from the skin surface [28] and the sebaceous glands between 0.5 and 2.7 mm from surface [18, 29].
- Injury to the sebaceous glands can result in obstruction and following pustule or cyst formation. Treat this with warm compresses to allow spontaneous drainage, or unroofing with a needle if persistent.
- Remember in patients with tighter scalps: The trichophytic closure widens the wound by cutting additional 1 mm. Sufficient scalp laxity must be available to allow trichophytic closure without causing excessive tension on the wound. When in doubt, it is much better to forego trichophytic closure than and create a slightly wider scar, than close the scalp tightly under tension and risk wound dehiscence.

Summary

FUT strip harvest is a time-tested technique for acquiring a large number of donor follicles in a relatively time and cost-efficient manner. Donor site closure results in a linear scar across the occipital and temporal scalp. This scar is generally not visible, even immediately postoperatively, if the hair is worn at least 1/2-inch long and scar visibility is further reduced with trichophytic closure techniques. Multiple hair transplants can be performed in the same patient with the FUT technique if further grafting is needed in the future. Additionally, the use of FUT for an initial transplant does not preclude the use of FUE harvest in future transplants. Excellent patient outcomes can be achieved with meticulous attention to detail during strip harvest, donor site closure, graft dissection, site preparation, and graft placement.

References

1. Willamson D, Gonzalez M, Finlay AY. The effect of hair loss on quality of life. J Eur Acad Dermatol Venereol. 2001;15(2):137–9.
2. Wells PA, Willmoth T, Russel RJ. Does fortune favour the bald? Psychological correlates of hair loss in males. Br J Psychol. 1995;86(pt 3):337–44.
3. Cash TF. Losing hair, losing points? The effects of male pattern baldness on social impression formation. J Appl Soc Psychol. 1990;20(2):154–67.
4. Tekiner H, Karamanou M. The forgotten hair transplantation experiment (1897) of Dr. Menahem Hodara (1869–1926). Indian J Dermatol Venereol Leprol. 2016;82(3):352–5.
5. Okuda S. The study of clinical experiments of hair transplantation. Jpn J Dermatolurol. 1939;46:135.
6. Orentreich N. Autografts in alopecia and other selected dermatologic conditions. Ann N Y Acad Sci. 1959;83:463–79.
7. Headington JT. Transverse microscopic anatomy of the human scalp. A basis for monomorphic approach to disorders of the hair follicle. Arch Dermatol. 1984;120:449–56.

8. Limmer BL. Elliptical donor stereoscopically assisted micrografting as an approach to further refinement in hair transplantation. J Dermatol Surg Oncol. 1994;20:789–93.
9. Unger W. Delineating the "safe" donor area for hair transplanting. Am J Cosmet Surg. 1994;11:239–43.
10. Rassman W, Bernstein R, McClellan R, Jones R. Follicular unit extraction: minimally invasive surgery for hair transplantation. Dermatol Surg. 2002;28:720–7.
11. Rousso D, Presti P. Follicular unit transplantation. Facial Plast Surg. 2008;24(4):381–8.
12. Bater KL, Ishii M, Joseph A, Su P, Nellis J, Ishii LE. Perception of hair transplant for androgenetic alopecia. JAMA Facial Plast Surg. 2016;18(6):413–8.
13. Abt NB, Quatela O, Heiser A, Jowett N, Tessler O, Lee LN. Association of hair loss with health utility measurement before and after hair transplant surgery in men and women. JAMA Facial Plast Surg. 2018;20(6):495–500.
14. Lee JA, Levy DA, Patel KG, Brennan E, Oyer SL. Hair transplantation in frontal fibrosing alopecia and lichen planopilaris: a systematic review. Laryngoscope. 2020; https://doi.org/10.1002/lary.28551. [Epub ahead of print].
15. Umaresan M, Mysore V. Controversies in hair transplantation. J Cutan Aesthet Surg. 2018;11:173–81.
16. Mayer T, Fleming RW. Aesthetic and reconstructive surgery of the scalp: Mosby Yearbook. St Louis: Mosby; 1992.
17. Kridel R, Liu E. Techniques for creating inconspicuous face-lift scars: avoiding visible incisions and loss of temporal hair. Arch Facial Plast Surg. 2003;5(4):325–33.
18. Marzola M. Trichophytic closure of donor area. Hair Transplant Forum Int. 2005;15:113–6.
19. Rose P. Overview of trichophytic closure. In: Unger W, editor. Hair transplant. New York: Thieme Medical Puglishers. 5th ed; 2005. p. 281–4.
20. Rose P. Ledge closure. Hair Transplant Forum Int. 2005;15:113–6.
21. Frechet P. Minimal scars for scalp surgery. J Dermatol Surg. 2007;33:45–56.
22. Lam S. Hair transplant 360: advances, techniques, business development, and global perspectives. Philadelphia: Jaypee Brother Med Publ Ltd.; 2015.
23. Mysore V. Hair transplantation. Philadelphia: Jaypee Brother Med Publ Ltd.; 2016.
24. Tan Baser N, Cigsar B, Balci Akbuga U, Terzioglu A, Aslan G. Follicular unit transplantation for male-pattern hair loss: evaluation of 120 patients. J Plast Reconstr Aesthet Surg. 2006;59(11):162–9.
25. Harris J. Follicular unit transplantation: dissecting and planting techniques. Facial Plast Surg Clin North Am. 2004;12(2):225–32.
26. Lam S. Hair transplant operative 360. In: Lam S, editor. Hair transplant 360 for physicians. 2nd ed. Philadelphia: Jaypee Brother Med Publ Ltd.; 2016.
27. Bernstein R, Rassman W. Follicular unit transplantation: 2005, issue on advanced cosmetic surgery. Dermatol Clin. 2005;23(3):393–414.
28. Jimenez F, Izeta A, Poblet E. Morphometric evaluation of human scalp hair follicle: practical implications for hair transplant surgeon and hair regeneration studies. Dermatol Surg. 2007;37:58–64.
29. Toll R, Jacobi U, Richter H, Lademann J, Schaefer H, Blume PU. Penetration profile of microspheres in follicular targeting of terminal hair follicles. J Invest Dermatol. 2004;123:168–76.

Follicular Unit Extraction Technique

7

Sahar Nadimi

Introduction

Grafting techniques have evolved over the years from the early use of large, 4-mm round punch grafts to the nearly exclusive use of follicular unit (FU) grafts, which is currently the preferred method for most surgical restorations [1]. FUs are naturally occurring groups of one to four terminal hairs in which all of the support structures—including sebaceous glands, subcutaneous fat, and a circumferential band of perifollicular collagen—remain intact (Fig. 7.1) [2]. The main problem associated with the use of larger grafts was related to the creation of an unnatural "doll's hair" or corn-row appearance. This deformity arose during wound healing as a result of circumferential contracture and compression of the graft's embedded hair follicles (Fig. 7.2). Compared with larger grafts, each of which contains multiple FUs and intervening skin, the final result following the strategic placement of individual FUs is a predictably natural appearance. Figure 7.3 shows the preoperative and postoperative views of a patient who underwent a total of 2988 follicular unit grafts to create a very natural and relatively dense appearance.

Follicular unit extraction (FUE) is a highly refined modification of traditional punch-graft harvesting that uses small circular punches to remove individual FUs from the donor area (Fig. 7.4) [3]. In recent years, FUE has become the fastest-growing procedure in hair restoration [4]. It was developed primarily to avoid the linear scar that accompanies elliptical strip harvesting. In contrast to strip scars, FU extraction sites heal with small, diffusely scattered circular scars that are often easier to camouflage for patients who prefer short hair lengths. This technique usually allows patients to cut their hair to approximately one-fourth inch or less. The

S. Nadimi (✉)
Department of Otolaryngology-Head and Neck Surgery,
Loyola University Medical Center, Maywood, IL, USA

Private Practice in Oakbrook Terrace, Maywood, IL, USA

© Springer Nature Switzerland AG 2020
L. N. Lee (ed.), *Hair Transplant Surgery and Platelet Rich Plasma*,
https://doi.org/10.1007/978-3-030-54648-9_7

Fig. 7.1 Hair grows on the scalp in follicular units, which appear as discrete bundles that generally contain one to four hairs each. The success of follicular unit grafting depends in the meticulous isolation of these units under high-power magnification

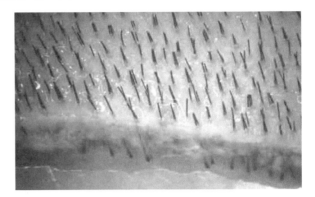

Fig. 7.2 Example of a "pluggy"-appearing hairline. The main problem associated with the use of larger grafts was related to the creation of an unnatural "doll's hair" or corn-row appearance. This deformity arose during wound healing as a result of circumferential contracture and compression of the graft's embedded hair follicles

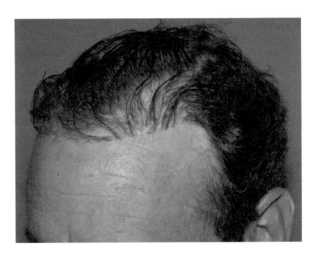

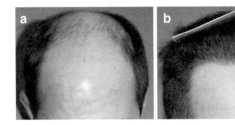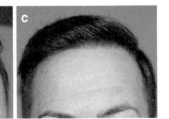

Fig. 7.3 Follicular unit hairline restoration. A total of 2988 grafts were used to create a very natural and relatively dense appearance in this patient with an advanced hair loss pattern. (**a**) Preoperative view. (**b**) Postoperative view with hair combed back. (**c**) Postoperative view

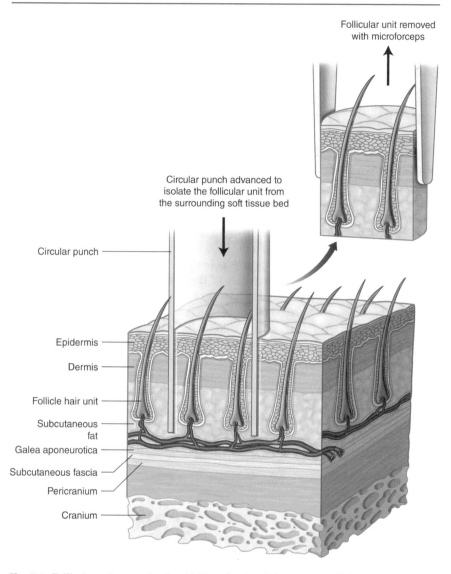

Follicular unit removed with microforceps

Circular punch advanced to isolate the follicular unit from the surrounding soft tissue bed

Circular punch

Epidermis

Dermis

Follicle hair unit

Subcutaneous fat

Galea aponeurotica

Subcutaneous fascia

Pericranium

Cranium

Fig. 7.4 Follicular unit extraction is a highly refined graft-harvesting technique that uses small circular punches that range between 0.8 and 1.2 mm in diameter to isolate individual follicular units. The epidermis is first scored to ensure that the unit is centered in the circular cut, and the punch is then advanced to isolate the unit from the surrounding soft tissue bed. The path of the hair shafts must be followed meticulously to avoid follicular transection. Once released from its attachment to the subcutaneous tissue, the follicular unit is gently grasped with microforceps and removed. (Modified from Cole [11]; and Konior and Gabel [12])

patient also benefits from less postoperative donor-site pain compared with strip harvesting. For patients who have decreased scalp laxity from prior strip harvesting procedures, follicular unit extraction may be performed to obtain additional grafts (assuming there is a sufficient donor hair supply) [5].

Indications for FUE

There are several indications for using FUE surgery (Table 7.1). In general, any patient who is a candidate for the strip method is a candidate for FUE, and the cosmetic results in the recipient area are the same for both surgeries. The most common candidates are those who desire the option of wearing their hair short after surgery. Patients, however, should be informed that there is no such thing as "scar-less surgery." Although there is no linear scarring, there will be small circular scars that will not allow most to shave their head after FUE surgery.

Another indication for FUE surgery is body hair harvest. FUE allows for the harvest of body hair without the creation of linear scars on the chest, abdomen, or submandibular areas. FUE can also be used to repair prior hair transplants. For example, inappropriately placed or linear hairlines, multihair grafts in the hairline, or visibly pluggy grafts can be repaired using FUE. In the case of a pluggy-appearing hairline due to multihair follicular units, the bulky grafts may be thinned by FUE [5]. Figure 7.5a shows a patient with a pluggy and unnatural-appearing hairline.

Table 7.1 Indications for FUE

1. Preference for short hair style
2. Tight donor region
3. Maximize donor capacity (FUE/strip combo procedures)
4. Hair transplant repair
   a. Debulking plugs and minigrafts
   b. Removal of undesirable hairline grafts
5. Body hair harvests

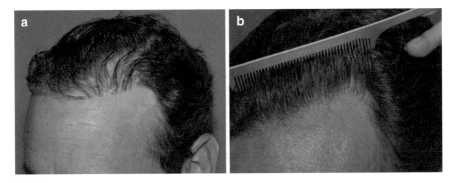

Fig. 7.5 Pluggy hairline repair. (**a**) A patient with a pluggy- and unnatural-appearing hairline. (**b**) The same patient who underwent repair of the pluggy hairline using FUE to debulk some of the larger grafts. Individual FUs were also placed in between the plugs to create a more natural- and dense-appearing hairline

Figure 7.5b shows the same patient who underwent repair of the pluggy hairline using FUE to debulk some of the larger grafts. Individual FUs were also placed in between the plugs to create a more natural- and dense-appearing hairline.

Donor Area Considerations

In general, the total number of grafts available using FUE is usually similar to the number available from strip harvesting, although the actual number is dependent on the density of the donor hair. The endpoint for FUE is thinning of the donor hair to a level that is visibly noticeable. It is crucial to avoid overharvesting in a small donor area, as this area may appear significantly less dense than the surrounding donor region, particularly if the patient wears a short haircut after surgery. A safe surgical plan is to distribute the FUE sites over the entire donor area (occipital and both temporal regions) at a uniform density relative to the native follicular unit density (Fig. 7.6).

FUE Punch Design

The major challenge in performing FUE is the uncertainty of the subcutaneous course and configuration of the follicles below the skin surface. These differences include the angulation, curvature, or splay of the follicles. Various FUE punches are

Fig. 7.6 FUE donor area. A safe surgical plan is to distribute the FUE sites over the entire donor area (occipital and both temporal regions) at a uniform density relative to the native follicular unit density

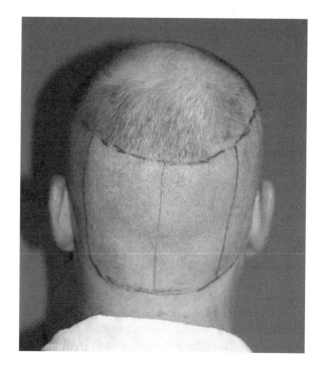

available to deal with these challenges. In general, there are three major categories of FUE punches: sharp, dull or blunt, and flat; within each category, there are manual and powered versions.

Sharp Punch Technique

Rassman and colleagues first described the sharp punch dissection and noted that follicle transection rates increased as dissection depths increased [3]. They advocated a limited-depth dissection to decrease follicle transection. In order to allow a more consistent depth of dissection, Cole developed a manual punch device with an adjustable mechanical depth limiter. A depth limiter, such as a bead or silicone tube on the punch, provides a physical barrier to skin entry. The limiter can be set at various depths, usually 2.0–2.5 mm, to allow graft removal. The punch is inserted, usually with a twisting motion in the case of a manual punch and directly into the skin using a powered punch. Grafts can be extracted by using a sharp punch to first score the skin and then to cut deep into the perifollicular fat. Maintaining a cutting location centered on the individual FU is crucial to avoid follicular transection. As previously mentioned, transection is a major concern with the sharp punches because the FU cannot be visualized as the punch penetrates into the donor scalp [1, 5].

A variety of manual sharp dermal punches are available, and the most common sizes for FUE are 0.8–1.0 mm. In general, patients with curlier hair follicles will require larger FUE punch sizes, whereas patients with straighter hair tend to allow for a smaller punch size. Although small punches are desirable for minimizing detectability of the residual circular scars, decreasing punch diameters increases the risk of transection by bringing the cutting edge closer to the target follicle.

The powered versions are also available from several hair restoration suppliers, such as the Neograft (Neograft Solutions, Dallas, TX) device, which has a suction apparatus that assists in harvesting and planting grafts.

Dull Punch Technique

The use of "dull" dissecting punches was developed for dealing with the unpredictable subcutaneous course and configuration of the follicles [5, 6]. The proposed mechanism is that the dull punch is less likely to cut the follicles and acts as a "guide" directing the follicles into the lumen of the punch. In addition to providing a low transection rate, a dull punch allows a deeper dissection that separates the follicles from the subcutaneous tissue.

In an attempt to reduce the risk of transection, a two-step process was developed that uses a sharp punch to first score the epidermis, followed by insertion of a dull dissecting punch to separate the FU from the deeper subcutaneous tissue [6]. Recent advances in FUE punch development have led to decreased follicular unit transection rates. The hybrid (flat) trumpet punch (WAW FUE Instruments©) is characterized by a 90 ° outer edge that makes penetration in the skin much less traumatic than the classic sharp punches. Once through the epidermis, its smooth funnel-shaped inner edge performs more of a dissection than a cutting role. The punch can then go deeper without damaging the hair follicles, which results in a decreased transection rate as compared to the traditional sharp punches.

Robotic FUE

Robotic devices are also available as an alternative to manual extraction to facilitate extracting larger numbers of FUs in a single session [7–10]. The robotic system was approved by the Food and Drug Administration for hair transplantation in 2011. The ARTAS System (Restoration Robotics, San Jose, CA) is a robotic device used under physician control [5]. The technique involves the placement of a skin tension device which stabilizes the skin. This skin tension device has fiducial markings on the periphery to define the donor region and provides data regarding the angles and directions of the hair follicles. The physician directs the robot to dissect random grafts a given distance apart, to select follicular units with a given number of hairs, or to dissect specific grafts that the physician selects.

Once the robot has selected a target graft, an inner sharp punch will initially penetrate or score the skin, just entering the epidermis, to a depth of approximately 1–2 mm. This is followed by a rotating dull punch that enters the skin to a greater depth to core out the graft and dissect the follicular unit free from the skin. Adjustments to the insertion depths of the two punches, the speed of rotation, and the angle of insertion are automated. The operator may make fine adjustments as needed during the dissection process. Once the system has completed the dissection with the skin tension device, it is moved to the next donor area and the process is repeated until the desired number of dissections has been completed. The follicular units are then removed from the donor area.

Performing the FUE Procedure

The donor-area hair is first shaved to 2–3 mm in length to help visualize the exit angle and direction of the protruding hair shafts. Depending on surgeon prefer-ence, the patient can be placed in a sitting or prone position. Local anesthesia with 0.5% lidocaine with 1:200,000 epinephrine is injected throughout the donor region. The punch is used to score the skin to ensure that the FU is centered in the middle of the circumferential cut. The punch is then carefully advanced using a rotary or oscillatory motion to isolate the FU from the surrounding soft-tissue bed. The path of the hair shafts must be followed meticulously to avoid follicular transection. Once released from its attachment to the subcutaneous tissue, the FU is gently grasped with microforceps and removed. This procedure is repeated until the desired number of grafts is obtained. Following their removal, the grafts are exam-ined under high-power magnification to ensure their integrity and to remove any

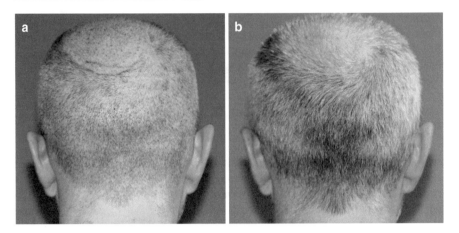

Fig. 7.7 FUE donor area. (**a**) The FUE donor area at postoperative day 4. (**b**) The same patient's donor area 3 weeks after FUE surgery

excess skin. Once the grafts have been dissected and removed from the donor area with care to avoid crush injury, they are immediately placed into the holding solution of choice.

Postoperative Care

Whether strip or FUE is performed, the recipient area is treated in a similar manner. An occlusive dressing and antibiotic ointment is applied over the donor area for the first night after surgery. Application of antibiotic ointment over the donor area is continued until the scabs over the extraction sites have been fully healed, which is usually achieved by postoperative days 5–7. Figure 7.7a shows the FUE donor area at postoperative day 4. Figure 7.7b shows the same patient's donor area 3 weeks after FUE surgery.

Summary

Follicular unit extraction (FUE) has become the fastest-growing procedure in hair restoration and is a valuable addition to the surgeon's repertoire. Many patients opt for FUE due to the excellent results, rapid recovery, and the ability to wear their hair short if they desire. FUE is also valuable in patients that require repairs and for former strip patients that require additional surgery. Recent advances in FUE punch development have led to decreased follicular transection rates and improved results.

References

1. Konior RJ, Nadimi S. Hair restoration. In: Flint PW, editor. Cummings otolaryngology: head & neck surgery. 7th ed. Philadelphia: Elsevier; In press. Chapter 22.
2. Bernstein RM, Rassman WR. The logic of follicular unit transplantation. Dermatol Clin. 1999;17:277.
3. Rassman WR, Bernstein RM, McClellan R, et al. Follicular unit extraction: minimally invasive surgery for hair transplantation. Dermatol Surg. 2002;28:720–8.
4. International Society of Hair Restoration Surgery. 2011 Practice census results, July 2011.
5. Harris JA. Follicular unit extraction. Facial Plast Surg Clin North Am. 2013;21:375–84.
6. Harris JA. Follicular unit extraction: the SAFE system. Hair Transplant Forum Int. 2004;14(157):163–4.
7. Harris JA. Powered blunt dissection with the SAFE system for FUE (part I and II). Hair Transplant Forum Int. 2010;20:188–9; 21:16–17, 2011.
8. Harris J. Robotic-assisted follicular unit extraction for hair restoration: case reports. Cosmet Dermatol. 2012;25:284–7.
9. Rose PT, Nusbaum B. Robotic hair restoration. Dermatol Clin. 2014;32(1):97–107.
10. Avram MR, Watkins SA. Robotic follicular unit extraction in hair transplantation. Dermatol Surg. 2014;40(12):1319–27.
11. Cole JP. An analysis of follicular punches, mechanics, and dynamics in follicular unit extraction. Facial Plast Surg Clin North Am. 2013;21:437–47.
12. Konior RJ, Gabel SP. Hair restoration: a sophisticated art form. Facial Plast Surg Clin North Am. 2013;21(3):xv–xvi.

Local Anesthesia and Scalp Blocks

8

Michael C. Lubrano, Chen Chen Costelloe, and Robert Jason Yong

Introduction

As most hair transplants are performed comfortably with only local anesthesia, understanding techniques including scalp nerve blocks and safety of local anesthesia medications is paramount. This chapter will cover the mechanism of action of local anesthetics, commonly used local anesthetics and their dosing, innervation of the skull, and how to block these peripheral nerves. Common complications from the use of local anesthetics are covered at the end of this chapter as well as how to manage them.

Local Anesthetics

Local anesthetics reversibly block the conduction of voltage-gated sodium channels and seize all nerve propagation, thus creating an environment conducive for both motor and sensory paralysis [1]. Peripheral sensory nerve blocks are essential to performing surgical procedures in the outpatient setting. The basic chemical structure of local anesthetics involves a tertiary amine and an aromatic ring that are connected via an amide or an ester bond. It is this specific bond that differentiates the two main classes of local anesthetics from one another. While function of these

M. C. Lubrano (✉)
South Shore Hospital, Department of Anesthesiology & Pain Medicine, South Weymouth, MA, USA

C. C. Costelloe
Brigham Healthcare, Department of Anesthesiology, Harvard Medical School, Boston, MA, USA

R. J. Yong
Division of Pain Medicine, Department of Anesthesiology and Pain Medicine, Brigham and Women's Hospital, Harvard Medical School, Boston, MA, USA

© Springer Nature Switzerland AG 2020
L. N. Lee (ed.), *Hair Transplant Surgery and Platelet Rich Plasma*,
https://doi.org/10.1007/978-3-030-54648-9_8

molecules remains the same, this bond differentiation has clinical significance when considering risk for allergic reactions, as we will discuss later in this chapter.

A number of factors influence the activity of local anesthetics These include anesthetic dose, the site of injection, and the injectate site pH. The dose and concentration of the local anesthetic will have the most pronounced effect on onset and duration of action. Also, injecting local anesthetic where the nerves have branched out will increase the surface area of nerve tissue exposed to local anesthetic, thus resulting in faster times of onset. The more basic the environment, the more molecules are able to cross the cell membrane and block neuronal action potential, resulting in a faster onset of action [3]. Sodium bicarbonate can therefore be used to increase the speed of onset by creating a more basic environment. Once the local attaches to the Na+ channel, it becomes charged and is much less likely to dissociate compared to their noncharged, hydrophobic form.

Commercially Used, Topical Local Anesthetics for Nerve Blocks

A myriad of local anesthetics are commercially available for use in clinical procedures and providers may choose nearly any local anesthetic for infiltration or peripheral nerve blocks. The most often-utilized amide agents include bupivacaine, lidocaine, mepivacaine, prilocaine, and ropivacaine. The ester local anesthetics used most commonly include chloroprocaine, procaine, and tetracaine. Pharmacologic properties of these drugs can be found in Table 8.1. A basic rule of thumb is that local anesthetics containing two "i's" in the name are amides versus those with one "i" which are esters.

Potency of a local anesthetic is depended on its *hydrophilicity*. Bupivacaine is more hydrophobic than lidocaine and thus less molecules needed to inhibit the action of Na+ channels [4]. Hydrophilic local anesthetics are, therefore, more potent, and less concentration of the drug is needed to achieve the desired effect when compared to less hydrophilic agents in this class.

The *onset time* of local anesthetic is depended on the *pKa* as well as the total dose injected. The pKa is the pH at which the local anesthetic will exist half in its

Table 8.1 Properties of common local anesthetics used for peripheral nerve blocks

Local anesthetic (brand name)	Bond type	Onset time	pKa	Max mg dose / kg	Max mg dose/ kg with epinephrine	Duration (hours)	Duration with epinephrine (hours)
Procaine	Ester	Fast	8.9	8	10	0.25–0.5	0.5–1
Chloroprocaine	Ester	Fast	9.1	10	15	0.25–0.5	0.5–1
Lidocaine	Amide	Fast	7.8	5	7	1–2	2–3
Mepivacaine	Amide	Fast	7.7	5	7	1–2	2–3
Prilocaine	Amide	Fast	8.0	7	8	1–2	2–3
Bupivacaine	Amide	Slow	8.1	2.0	2.5	3–6	4–7
Ropivacaine	Amide	Slow	8.07	3	3	3–6	4–7

Adapted from [2] and [4]

Table 8.2 Commercially available local anesthetics and brands

Generic name	Brand name	Common concentration (%)
Procaine	Novocaine	1–2
Chloroprocaine	Nesacaine	1–2
Lidocaine	Xylocaine	0.5–1
Mepivacaine	Carbocaine	0.5–1
Prilocaine	Citanest	0.5–1
Bupivacaine	Marcaine	0.25–0.5
Ropivacaine	Naropin	0.25–0.5

Adapted from [2]

lipid-soluble (uncharged) and half in its water-soluble (charged) form. pKa determines how much of the drug charged versus uncharged when entering an anticipated pH of around 7.4 in humans. For example, lidocaine has a pKa of 7.8, one of the local anesthetics that is closest to a 50:50 lipophilic to hydrophilic ratio at physiologic pH, contributing to its almost immediate fast onset. The closer the drug's pKa to physiological pH, the faster the onset.

The *duration of action* for local anesthetics is dependent on *protein binding*. Ropivacaine and bupivacaine, for example, are highly protein bound, and therefore, their duration of action is longer.

In general, most proceduralists will inject lidocaine with epinephrine (1:200,000) to quickly anesthetize an anatomic area for fast interventions. This can be combined with longer acting locals to provide a longer lasting block. One benefit of longer lasting local anesthetics is that the patient may experience longer pain relief after they leave the procedural site. Bupivacaine and ropivacaine are long-acting local anesthetics of choice for peripheral nerve blocks because of their relative safety, commercial availability, and several hours duration. Bupivacaine and ropivacaine have similar potencies although ropivacaine is considered to be less cardiotoxic. Either of these medications can be injected with epinephrine to reduce systemic absorption and extend the duration of the block. Common concentrations of local anesthetics used for nerve blocks are 2% lidocaine, 0.5% ropivacaine, and bupivacaine. Ropivacaine, as a reference, costs greater than 10 times more than bupivacaine (Table 8.2).

Max Doses

The math to calculate maximum doses can be confusing and daunting because the max doses are listed in milligrams per kilogram and the local anesthetics are dosed in milliliters with differing concentrations.

The first step is to convert the local anesthetic concentration to milligrams per milliliter by multiplying the concentration by 10. This will *always* convert a medication listed as a percent into mg/ml. For example, bupivacaine 0.25% would be $0.25 \times 10 = 2.5$ mg/ml. Lidocaine 1% would be $1 \times 10 = 10$ mg/ml.

Now, the calculation of allowable milliliters can be calculated based on the chart. For example, lidocaine with epinephrine max dose is 7 mg/kg, which would be 490 mg for a 70-kg adult; 490 mg would be 49 ml of 1% lidocaine with epinephrine.

Another example with bupivacaine 0.25% with epinephrine would equal 2.5 mg/ml, with a max dose of 2.5 mg/kg, a 70-kg adult would be able to receive 70 kg * 2.5 mg/kg = 175 mg/2.5 mg/ml = 70 ml. *Therefore, an easy way to calculate the max dose of bupivacaine 0.25% with epinephrine is to take their weight in kg and convert it 1:1 into ml.* Doubling the concentration of bupivacaine to 0.5% would require half the dose, so a 70-kg adult would be able to receive 35 ml of bupivacaine.

Local anesthetic	Maximum dose/kg (mg/kg)	Calculated dose (mg)	Maximum volume (ml)
Lidocaine 1% plain	4	280	28
Lidocaine 1% with epi	7	490	49
Bupivacaine 0.25%	2.5	175	70
Bupivacaine 0.5%	2.5	175	35

When using more than one local anesthetic, the max dose is cumulative and must be calculated carefully. For example, in the 70-kg adult receiving lidocaine 1% with epinephrine, the max dose is 49 ml. If the surgeon uses 25 ml of the lidocaine to infiltrate the incision and wants to use bupivacaine for scalp blocks, the patient has already received 50% of the max dose of lidocaine so is only able to receive 50% of the max dose of bupivacaine. In this example, the 70-kg adult can only receive 35 ml of bupivacaine 0.25% with epinephrine in addition to the lidocaine used previously.

If performing hair transplantation with a scalp block, bupivacaine 0.25% with epinephrine can be used which would require 15–20 ml. This would represent 20–25% of the max dose, thus allowing 75% of the max dose of lidocaine to be used to infiltrate the donor site and recipient field using lidocaine 1% with epinephrine which would be roughly 35 ml in the 70-kg adult.

Adjuvants for Local Anesthetics Injections

Medications may be added to local anesthetic solutions to increase the duration and potency of the block. The most common additive found in local anesthetic is epinephrine. Epinephrine acts as a vasoconstrictor when injected in the subcutaneous tissue. Epinephrine has been shown to prolong peripheral nerve blocks for some local anesthetics, particularly when used in conjunction with lidocaine or mepivacaine [5]. The vasoconstrictive properties of epinephrine limit the amount of local anesthetic that is absorbed systemically. This allows for an increase in the total weight-based dose of the local anesthetic that may be used at any given time. Local with epinephrine use should be used with caution in patients with severe cardiovascular disease or other disease states with presumed, tenuous hemodynamic statuses such as untreated hyperthyroidism and hypertension.

- *Epinephrine should be used with caution in patients with tenuous cardiovascular status or other diseases with labile hemodynamic status such as untreated hyperthyroidism or hypertension.*

Sensory Innervation of the Scalp

Several, primary nerves are responsible for the cutaneous, sensory innervation of the scalp. These can be separated into three major categories: the anterior, lateral, and posterior regions. Trigeminal nerve terminal branches innervate the anterior region of the scalp. As the ophthalmic division of the trigeminal nerve travels through the superior orbital fissure above the eye, it separates into three distinct nerves: the nasociliary, lacrimal, and the frontal [6]. It is the frontal nerve that ultimately splits into the two nerves in this region that require anesthetizing: the supraorbital and supratrochlear nerves (Fig. 8.1).

- The *supraorbital nerve* enters the subcutaneous facial tissue above each eye via the superior orbital foramen. This is located at the mid pupillary line just below the supraorbital ridge.
- The *supratrochlear nerve* is located medial to this and traverses over the supraorbital ridge superiorly as well. These two nerves are responsible for cutaneous innervation of the medial and upper eyelid as well as the anterolateral forehead extending to the top of the scalp.
- The *zygomaticotemporal nerve* is a terminal branch of the zygomatic nerve, which exits through a small outlet at the level of the lateral canthus behind the orbital rim [6].
- The *auriculotemporal nerve* is a branch of the mandibular nerve. One can trace its path by identifying the parotid gland and the area anterior to the tragus of the

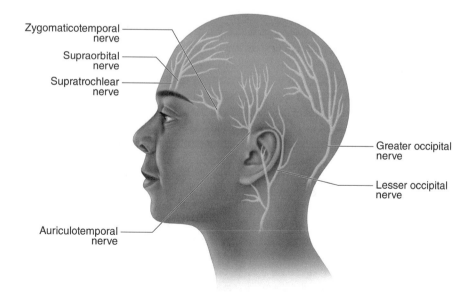

Fig. 8.1 Innervation of the scalp

ear. This nerve begins in the parotid gland and travels to supply sensation over the temporomandibular joint and external auditory meatus before running superiorly in parallel to the temporal artery until reaching the superior aspect of the lateral scalp [7]. Overall, the cutaneous innervation includes the lateral canthus and temporal region as well as the region anterior to the auricle extending superiorly up the side of the scalp.

The occipital nerves provide the innervation for the posterior aspect of the scalp and are divided into three branches: the greater, lesser, and third occipital nerves.

- The *greater occipital nerve* is a terminal branch of the dorsal ramus of C2, and it exits the skull alongside the occipital artery at the level of the superior nuchal ridge [6]. This is approximately one third of the distance between the occipital protuberance and the mastoid process when moving laterally.
- The *lesser occipital nerve* originates from the second and third cervical nerves. It travels posterior to the sternocleidomastoid muscle and extends superiorly in order to innervate the scalp just inferiorly and laterally to the grater occipital nerve [7].
- The third occipital nerve innervates the lower occipital aspect of the posterior region of the scalp. This nerve is a terminal branch of C3. It is not recommended that this nerve be blocked without ultrasound guidance because vertebral vessels course below this area [8].

Techniques for Blocking Regions of the Scalp

The smallest needle should be used such as a 25- or 30-gauge needle. A licensed provider must assess the appropriateness of any nerve block for every patient prior to proceeding with any procedure. This includes reviewing a patient's medical history for any medication allergies, anatomic aberrancy or trauma around intended location sites, and the presence of any cutaneous or subcutaneous infections. The desired area should be sterilized with alcohol before local injection. The entire scalp can be blocked with approximately 15–20 ml of 0.25% bupivacaine or ropivacaine.

During the injection, the needle will penetrate the skin, subcutaneous tissue, and aponeurosis before encountering the periosteum. Once the needle is inserted into the proper location, one must aspirate prior to placement of the local anesthetic to ensure that the needle is not intravascular. While the tip of the needle is in contact with periosteum, the injectate will spread along the loose connective tissue plane. After the needle is withdrawn, direct pressure over the injectate will spread the injectate along the loose connective tissue plane and allow for diffusion to the targeted nerves located in the aponeurosis. The targets for injection will be away from the trunk of the nerves to decrease likelihood of neurovascular puncture and damage. By avoiding the trunk, the target is also where the nerves are desiccating, thus increasing the surface area of the injected nerve resulting in a quicker onset. This technique for injecting minimizes the need to fan the needle while still achieving adequate spread and coverage.

To block the anterior region of the scalp involve two sites:

1. Identify the supraorbital notch, a small groove located superior and medial to the margin of the orbit, and the frontal bone, superior along the mid-pupillary line. Insert the needle (smallest gauge available) one fingerbreadth above the brow perpendicular to the forehead and advance the needle until bone is contacted. While maintaining contact with periosteum with a beveled needle, inject approximately 1 ml of local anesthetic superficial to the periosteum into the loose connective tissue plane. Remove the needle and spread the injectate by applying pressure to flatten out the local anesthetic. Repeat on the contralateral side, and this will anesthetize the supraorbital nerves.
2. Insert a needle one fingerbreadth or 1 cm midline to the supraorbital injection site and inject 1 ml of local anesthetic. After applying pressure, this should effectively block the supratrochlear nerves [8] which run just lateral to midline.

Blocking the lateral aspect of the scalp involves two steps:

1. Identify the posterior aspect of the lateral orbital rim. To anesthetize the zygomaticotemporal nerve, insert a needle one fingerbreadth above the brow superior to the lateral orbital rim and inject 1–2 ml of local anesthetic.
2. To anesthetize the auriculotemporal nerve [8], insert the needle one fingerbreadth above the ear superior to the tragus and inject 2 ml of local anesthetic.

There are several techniques to block the greater and lesser occipital nerves. One option is to make a long subcutaneous wheel along the nuchal line. Another way is to identify the superior nuchal line approximately one third of the distance moving laterally from the occipital protuberance to the mastoid process. The needle should be inserted just medial to the occipital artery, which can be identified via manual palpation at this level and directed in a perpendicular angle until it reaches bone. An alternative method is to first find the midpoint between the crown of the head and the occipital protuberance midline. Then, take the midpoint between the found point and the mastoid process and inject 2 ml of local anesthetic. This alternative method will target the desiccating greater occipital nerves.

The lesser occipital nerve is blocked by one of the two ways. The first is done by slightly retracting the needle after completing the greater occipital nerve block to just below the skin and redirecting it inferiorly and laterally [8] and injecting 2 ml of local anesthetic. The second is by inserting the needle inferior and posterior to the mastoid process and injecting 2 ml of local anesthetic.

Local Anesthetic Allergies, Toxicity, and Management

The total amount of local anesthetic absorbed systemically is directly proportional to the dose injected into the original anatomic site of interest. Other important factors responsible for systemic absorption include injectate volume, site of infiltration, local anesthetic molecular properties, and the presence of a vasocon-strictor [9]. As previously discussed, 5 µg/ml of epinephrine added to any solution can significantly decrease the incidence of systemic toxicity when utilizing safe doses of anesthetic.

Once administered, local anesthetics are rapidly distributed throughout the body and in every type of bodily tissues as they become absorbed. Aminoamide class of locals is mainly metabolized in the liver while esters are broken down in the plasma by pseudocholinesterase. A major product of ester (only one "i") metabolism is para-aminobenzoic acid (PABA), a compound responsible for allergic reactions. Hypersensitivity to amides is rarer compared to esters. Numerous other preservatives such as methylparaben, paraben, or sulfites may also trigger IgE-mediated reactions in patients.

True type I hypersensitivity reactions to local anesthetics are found in less than 1% of patients [10]. There are more documented cases with amide anesthetics; however, this is likely due to the greater prevalence of the use of these drugs. Despite these concerns, allergic reactions to local anesthetics are exceedingly rare. Immunology clinics that routinely receive patient referrals with suspected local anesthetic allergy often find that the great majority do not have true allergies after comprehensively testing [11]. This suggests that many of the preservatives are potentially responsible for allergic events. When a patient begins to experience signs and symptoms of allergic reaction peri-procedurally, the treatment is generally supportive. If symptoms are minimal, such as hives, then stopping the procedure and simply administering diphenhydramine is appropriate. If allergic symptoms progress to trouble breathing or hypotension suggestive of anaphylaxis or anaphylactoid reaction, a code blue should be activated; administration of 100% oxygen, intramuscular epinephrine, and steroids would be recommended as well as transfer to a nearby emergency department for further management.

LAST or local anesthetic systemic toxicity is one of the most feared complications of local injection. Toxicity due to its action on voltage-gated Na+ channels, particularly in the brain and the myocardium [10] when the recommended dose is exceeded. The symptoms and physiologic effects of LAST are detailed in Table 8.3. Prodromal symptoms include symptoms like altered mental status, tinnitus, and

Table 8.3 Local anesthetic systemic toxicity (LAST)

Symptoms	Physiologic effects
Dysphoria	Dyspnea
Altered mental status	Chest pain
Tinnitus	Seizure
Metallic taste	Bradycardia or tachycardia
Dysarthria	Hypotension or hypertension
Perioral numbness	Ventricular arrhythmias
Auditory disturbances	Asystole

Adapted from [12]

perioral numbness. These symptoms precipitate within minutes of local anesthetic injection in about 20% of these patients before progressing to more concerning, systemic effects. LAST can lead to life-threatening hemodynamic collapse; hence, it must be identified and treated rapidly.

It is imperative that clinicians follow an office-based emergency protocol for assessing and supporting the patient whenever LAST is suspected. Table 8.4 lists a series of recommended steps to follow in the instance of a LAST occurrence [12]. Immediate actions involve calling for help, acquiring a code cart, serial vital signs, and providing 100% oxygen to the patient. It is possible that patient may seize as a result of local anesthetics on the brain. Seizures can be treated with IV benzodiazepines such as midazolam. The most important medication to have immediately available in any procedure area where local anesthetics are used is lipid emulsion, also known as Intralipid. Lipid emulsion comprises 20% lipid that acts as a lipid sink in the plasma to bind local anesthetics. Rapid administration of a 1.5 mg/kg IV bolus of this medication is the immediate treatment of choice followed by an infusion of 0.25 ml/kg/min until the return of cardiovascular function.

- Lipid emulsion comprises 20% lipid that acts as a lipid sink in the plasma to bind local anesthetics.
- Rapid administration of a 1.5 mg/kg IV bolus of this medication is the immediate treatment of choice for LAST followed by an infusion of 0.25 ml/kg/min until the return of cardiovascular function.

Table 8.4 Local anesthetic toxicity management protocol

Step	Actions
1. Activate emergency protocol	Call for help
	Alert staff to make emergency cart available
	Request that lipid emulsion (Intralipid) be brought to bedside
	Have staff notify external facilities or hospitals that can provide advanced care
2. Immediate supportive care	Provide 100% oxygen by facemask
	In the event of seizure, administer benzodiazepines
3. Initiate life support	ACLS preferred
	Minimize epinephrine doses
	Avoid cardiovascular suppressing medications
4. Provide lipid emulsion (Intralipid) therapy	Lipid emulsion bolus of 1.5 ml/kg IV given rapidly over 1 min
	Follow with lipid emulsion infusion 0.25 ml/kg/min
	If hemodynamically unstable, one may repeat initial bolus 1–2 times and double infusion rate
	Maintain infusion for several minutes beyond patient stabilization
5. Transfer patient	Unstable patients require transfer to external facility for advanced care
	In cases of hemodynamic collapse, ECMO is indicated

Adapted from [12]

Conclusion

Successfully anesthetizing the scalp for interventional procedures requires an appropriate knowledge of anatomy as well as the pharmacokinetics and pharmacodynamics of the local anesthetics used. Local anesthetics impede the pain stimuli signaling by inhibiting the Na+ channels of peripheral nerves. The most commonly used medications for these blocks include lidocaine 1% with 1:100,000 or 1:200,000 epinephrine and ropivacaine or bupivacaine 0.25% with 1:200,000 or 1:400,000 epinephrine. It is also important to have appropriate emergency medications and equipment to effectively treat any unwanted complication that may arise from the use of local anesthetics. This includes allergic reactions as well as lipid emulsion (Intralipid), which is the only definitive therapy for local anesthetic systemic toxicity (LAST).

References

1. Enna SJ, Bylund DB. Elsevier Science (Firm). XPharm: the comprehensive pharmacology reference: Elsevier; 2008. https://www-sciencedirect-com.ezproxy.lib.uconn.edu/reference-work/9780080552323/xpharm-the-comprehensive-pharmacology-reference. Accessed 5 Nov 2018.
2. Berde CB, Strichartz GR. Chapter 36: Local anesthetics. In: Miller RD, Cohen NH, Fleisher LA, Wiener-Kronish JP, Young WL, editors. Miller's anesthesia eighth edition. Eight. Philadelphia: Elsevier Saunders; 2015. p. 2029–1055.
3. Wong K, Strichartz GR, Raymond SA. On the mechanisms of potentiation of local anesthetics by bicarbonate buffer: drug structure-activity studies on isolated peripheral nerve. Anesth Analg. 1993;76(1):131–43. http://www.ncbi.nlm.nih.gov/pubmed/8418714. Accessed 5 Nov 2018.
4. Becker DE, Reed KL. Essentials of local anesthetic pharmacology. Anesth Prog. 2006;53(3):98–108; quiz 109-10. https://doi.org/10.2344/0003-3006(2006)53[98:EOLAP]2.0.CO;2.
5. Kirksey MA, Haskins SC, Cheng J, Liu SS. Local anesthetic peripheral nerve block adjuvants for prolongation of analgesia: a systematic qualitative review. Schwentner C, ed. PLoS One. 2015;10(9):e0137312. https://doi.org/10.1371/journal.pone.0137312.
6. Dalley AF, Agur AM, editors. Clinically oriented anatomy. Philadelphia: Lippincott Williams & Wilkins; 2018.
7. Erdine S, Racz GB, Noe CE. Somatic blocks of the head and neck. In: Loeser JD, Manchikanti L, Sluijter ME, editors. Interventional pain management: image-guided procedures. 2nd ed. Philadelphia: Saunders Elsevier; 2008. p. 77–107.
8. Davies T, Karanovic S, Shergill B. Essential regional nerve blocks for the dermatologist: part 1. Clin Exp Dermatol. 2014;39(7):777–84. https://doi.org/10.1111/ced.12427.
9. Tucker GT. Pharmacokinetics of local anaesthetics. Br J Anaesth. 1986;58(7):717–31. http://www.ncbi.nlm.nih.gov/pubmed/3524638. Accessed 7 Nov 2018.
10. Liu W, Yang X, Li C, Mo A. Adverse drug reactions to local anesthetics: a systematic review. Oral Surg Oral Med Oral Pathol Oral Radiol. 2013;115(3):319–27. https://doi.org/10.1016/j.oooo.2012.04.024.
11. Kvisselgaard AD, Mosbech HF, Fransson S, Garvey LH. Risk of immediate-type allergy to local anesthetics is overestimated—results from 5 years of provocation testing in a Danish Allergy Clinic. J Allergy Clin Immunol Pract. 2018;6(4):1217–23. https://doi.org/10.1016/j.jaip.2017.08.010.
12. Park KK, Sharon VR. A review of local anesthetics. Dermatol Surg. 2017;43(2):173–87. https://doi.org/10.1097/DSS.0000000000000887.

Postoperative Expectations and Instructions

9

Samuel L. Oyer

Introduction

The success of any aesthetic procedure, such as surgical hair transplant, rests on numerous factors, including patient selection, surgical technique, and postoperative care. Surgeons often focus heavily on the details involved in surgical planning and technique, but may devote less attention to preparing their patients for what to expect in the postoperative period. A masterfully performed surgical procedure can be quickly derailed by improper postoperative care of the surgical site. Additionally, a patient who is incompletely informed about postoperative expectations may view normal portions of their recovery in a negative light, which risks undermining their satisfaction with an otherwise technically successful surgery. Particularly in a procedure such as hair transplant, where success is defined as much by subjective patient satisfaction as by quantitative hair growth, the surgeon should ensure that each patient has a clear and complete understanding of what to expect during the postoperative recovery. As is often stated with the care of a surgical patient, a surgeon who discusses potential surgical risks and complications prior to surgery is providing informed consent, but a surgeon who has this discussion after surgery is providing excuses.

The final results of hair transplant surgery are not seen for at least 1 year after surgery, so for many patients, the postoperative relationship with their surgeon lasts much longer than their preoperative relationship. Therefore, it is critical that the surgeon provides each patient with a detailed understanding of postoperative expectations during the recovery period. This is usually best accomplished by providing patients with detailed written instructions prior to their surgery along with verbal reinforcement of these instructions as needed during recovery. It is also critical that

S. L. Oyer (✉)
Facial Plastic & Reconstructive Surgery, University of Virginia, Charlottesville, VA, USA
e-mail: oyer@musc.edu

© Springer Nature Switzerland AG 2020
L. N. Lee (ed.), *Hair Transplant Surgery and Platelet Rich Plasma*,
https://doi.org/10.1007/978-3-030-54648-9_9

all office staff members who patients may encounter are up-to-date and informed on the postoperative wound care instructions and expectations, so patients receive consistent instructions for their postoperative questions or concerns. It cannot be overstated that providing patients with easy access to you and your staff during recovery, via telephone and in-person visits, is vital to ensuring patient confidence and satisfaction during recovery from a procedure that requires a significant amount of trust in the surgeon when results are delayed by months to years. Patient dissatisfaction, and correspondingly the risk of litigation [1, 2], is much higher when patients feel that their concerns are dismissed or they do not have adequate access to their medical providers.

There are very few data to guide the surgeon when providing patients with postoperative instructions, so specific recommendations will vary based on a surgeon's individual experience and training. Future studies specifically evaluating the role of postoperative medication regimens including steroids, antibiotics, analgesics, and topical biologics will help guide surgeons' use of these therapies in an evidence-based fashion. The following recommendations are meant as general guidelines to educate patients regarding recovery following hair transplant surgery. These recommendations are most easily organized in a timeline fashion with clear and concise instructions provided as a printed handout to patients [3].

Prior to Surgery

- *Medications*
  - Avoid Nonsteroidal anti-inflammatory drugs (NSAIDs) and certain herbals (Echinacea, garlic, ginkgo biloba, ginseng) that increase bleeding risk for 7 days prior to surgery.
  - The need to stop prescription anticoagulants should be discussed with the prescribing provider and the benefits/risks associated should be reviewed on an individual patient basis.
  - There are limited data that persistent bleeding related to continuing prescription anticoagulation use through hair transplant does not negatively affect graft survival [4].
  - Topical minoxidil (Rogaine®) containing products should be stopped 1 week prior to surgery.
  - Oral finasteride (Propecia©) should be continued during the entire perioperative period.
- *Activity*
  - Stop all nicotine containing products 2–4 weeks prior to the surgery [5, 6].
  - Avoid consuming alcohol 2–7 days prior to surgery to limit excessive bleeding.
- *Grooming*
  - Keep occipital hair at least 1–2 inches long if undergoing Follicular unit transfer (FUT) transplant to hide the suture line postoperatively.
  - For patients who color their hair, they should do so within 1 week of the procedure, so hair color is maintained in the early postoperative period.

Day of Surgery

- Shower and wash hair with antimicrobial soap the morning of surgery but do not apply any styling products to the hair.
- If IV sedation is not used, the patient is encouraged to eat a light breakfast prior to surgery.
- The patient should wear comfortable, loosing fitting clothing including a button-down shirt that does not need to be pulled over the head.

After Surgery

- *Medications*
  - Prescription opioid/acetaminophen analgesics are taken every 4–6 hours as needed. Individual opioid tolerance will vary among patients, but typically for opioid naïve patients, no more than 5–6 tablets will be required.
  - Patients may resume NSAID pain medication starting 48 hours after surgery.
  - Prophylactic antibiotics effective against skin flora such as cephalexin may be given for 3–5 days to prevent infection. Although hair transplant is considered a clean rather than sterile procedure, infection rates are very low and further study may demonstrate limited benefit from postoperative systemic antibiotics. Data regarding the use of routine systemic prophylactic antibiotics in facial plastic surgeries are mixed [7–9], and careful antibiotic stewardship should always be weighed against the risk of infection in each patient.
  - Oral corticosteroids may be prescribed for 3–5 days after transplant to help limit edema of the forehead that is common after graft placement and usually peaks 2–4 days after transplant [10]. The use of corticosteroids has not been specifically studied following hair transplant, and there is no universally accepted dosing regimen, but several authors suggest that faster resolution of forehead edema is seen with corticosteroid use [3, 10, 11].
  - Topical minoxidil (Rogaine®) containing products may be resumed 1 week following surgery. Topical minoxidil is helpful at the donor and recipient site to limit postoperative shedding and shock loss.
  - Oral finasteride (Propecia©) should be continued during the entire perioperative period.
  - The newly transplanted grafts must be kept moist as they are healing to allow for adequate oxygenation and vascularization. Topical saline spray should be applied gently to the recipient sites every 1–2 hours for the first 48 hours after surgery. The patient is given a spray bottle at the end of the procedure and asked to use it regularly until the bottle is empty. There is some evidence that the addition of liposomal adenosine triphosphate (ATP) to the saline spray may improve graft survival by providing the free grafts a usable energy source in the form of ATP, but this is not routinely used by all surgeons [12].
  - Topical antibiotic ointment such as bacitracin or surgical lubricant is applied to the donor-site sutures twice a day until the sutures are removed.

- *Activity*
  - Patients should sleep with their head elevated 15–30 degrees in the first week after surgery to minimize swelling.
  - Patients should avoid heavy lifting, strenuous activity, and bending at the waist for 1 week after surgery to avoid disrupting grafts. It takes about 4 days before any substantial wound healing has occurred to anchor the new grafts in place.
  - Ice can be placed on the forehead (not the implanted grafts) gently for 20 minutes every hour for the first 2–3 days to reduce forehead swelling.
  - Should grafts dislodge, the patient may recover them and bring them immediately to the office on saline-moistened gauze. If the grafts appear well hydrated, re-implantation may be attempted, but the patient should be warned that these grafts may not survive fully.
  - Slight bleeding from the recipient sites is common in the first 1–2 days after surgery and should be managed with gentle pressure using a clean damp gauze.
  - Patients may resume normal activity after 7 days, but in particularly tight scalps, consideration should be given to minimizing neck flexion for 4–6 weeks to limit stress on donor-site closure for FUT transplant.
- *Grooming*
  - Showering is permitted 24 hours after surgery by gently applying shampoo over the graft sites, allowing this to set for 2–3 minutes and gently rinsing by pouring water from a pitcher or gentle shower spray. Dandruff shampoo may help minimize itching. The grafts should be dried gently by dabbing with gauze or paper towel as regular terrycloth towels may adhere to the grafts. Combing the hair should be done only when the hair is wet and gently with fingers without contacting the scalp to avoid manipulating the grafts.
  - After the first day, the hair should be shampooed twice a day as described above. Small crusts commonly form around the grafts, and these should not be disrupted manually, but allowed to lift off by naturally. Most crusting ceases by 7–10 days after surgery. Gentle combing may be performed 3–5 days after surgery as long as the scalp is not contacted. A hair dryer on low setting may also be used starting 3 days after surgery to help dry the hair.
  - Hair products may be used starting 7 days after surgery, but patients should take care that hairspray does not directly contact the scalp. Spraying a comb with hairspray then combing the hair may be more effective.
  - The hair surrounding the grafts may be cut or colored starting 2 weeks after surgery.
  - Folliculitis commonly occurs at the recipient sites and should be managed by warm compresses several times per day or manual unroofing of persistent pustules with a needle. Rarely are topical antibiotic ointments required.
- *Follow-up*
  - When feasible, a short-term follow-up 1–2 days after the transplant is advised. This allows the surgeon to carefully evaluate the donor and recipient sites to ensure adequate adherence to postoperative instructions and to help address patient concerns about their early recovery.

- For FUT harvest, sutures are usually removed 7–10 days following surgery. Additional assessment of the grafts is performed at this time, and the patient is reminded of the postoperative course and risk for postoperative shedding.
- Intermediate follow-up to assess short-term hair growth around 6 months after surgery can evaluate early growth, patient adherence to continued medical regimen, and donor-site healing.
- Long-term follow-up at 1 year and beyond should be done to assess final graft survival and overall success of the transplant along with patient satisfaction of the results. Additional questions or plans for further treatment may be pursued at this time.

Postoperative Expectations

One of the most critical aspects of recovering from hair transplant that should be discussed with patients is the time frame for final results. Due to the timing of the hair growth cycle, new hair growth following transplant takes a while to manifest. Patients should be informed that new hair growth *begins* around 3–6 months after transplant with full growth achieved anywhere from 9 to 14 months and final success should not be evaluated until at least *1 year* from transplant [11]. Another important risk that should be carefully explained is the risk of postoperative shock loss that can occur at the recipient or donor site following transplant. This may be related to a combination of anagen and telogen effluvium and female patients or those with extensive miniaturization seem to be at highest risk [12]. This type of hair loss is quite alarming to patients if they are not prepared, but they should be informed that it is not permanent loss. Typically, shock loss begins 2–6 weeks following the procedure, and recovery starts by 3 months but can take up to 8 months to recover. Topical minoxidil use in the postoperative period can help minimize the extent of this loss [13].

Summary

Hair transplantation is a very effective procedure with high patient satisfaction, but this satisfaction is based on the patient's subjective evaluation of the entire process that includes the surgical transplant along with a minimum of 1 year of follow-up. The successful hair transplant surgeon should focus on excellent patient care and communication throughout this entire process. Time devoted prior to surgery preparing patients with what to expect after surgery pays dividends toward improving the physician–patient relationship and improving patient satisfaction. Postoperative instructions should specifically cover medication usage, wound care, activity restrictions, grooming habits, and timeframe for various stages of healing.

References

1. Svider PF, Keeley BR, Zumba O, Mauro AC, Setzen M, Eloy JA. From the operating room to the courtroom: a comprehensive characterization of litigation related to facial plastic surgery procedures. Laryngoscope. 2013;123(8):1849–53.
2. Vincent C, Young M, Phillips A. Why do people sue doctors? A study of patients and relatives taking legal action. Lancet. 1994;343(8913):1609–13.
3. Lam S. Hair Transplant Operative. In: Lam S, editor. Hair Transplant 360 for Physicians. 2nd ed. Philadelphia: Jaypee Brother Med Publ Ltd; 2016. p. 360.
4. Seong GH, Lee DY, Kim MH, Park BC. Excessive and persistent local bleeding at the hair transplant site of a patient taking warfarin and its effect on hair survival. Dermatol Surg. 2019; https://doi.org/10.1097/DSS.0000000000002190. [Epub ahead of print].
5. Sorensen LT. Wound healing and infection in surgery: the pathophysiological impact of smoking, smoking cessation, and nicotine replacement therapy: a systematic review. Ann Surg. 2012;255(6):1069–79.
6. Coon D, Tuffaha S, Christensen J, Bonawitz SC. Plastic surgery and smoking: a prospective analysis of incidence, compliance, and complications. Plast Reconstr Surg. 2013;131(2):385–91.
7. Gonzalez-Castro J, Lighthall JG. Antibiotic use in facial plastic surgery. Facial Plast Surg Clin North Am. 2016;24(30):347–56.
8. Ishii LE, Tollefson TT, Basura GJ, et al. Clinical practice guideline: improving nasal form and function after rhinoplasty executive summary. Otolaryngol Head Neck Surg. 2017;156(2):205–19.
9. Olds C, Spataro E, Li K, Kandathil C, Most SP. Postoperative antibiotic use among patients undergoing functional facial plastic and reconstructive surgery. JAMA Facial Plast Surg. 2019;21(6):491–7.
10. Konoir RJ. Complications in hair-restoration surgery. Facial Plast Surg Clin North Am. 2013;21(3):505–20.
11. Avram M, Rogers N. Contemporary hair transplantation. Dermatol Surg. 2009;35:1705–19.
12. Rose PT. Advances in hair restoration. Dermatol Clin. 2018;36(1):57–62.
13. True RH, Dorin RJ. A protocol to prevent shock loss. Hair Transplant Forum Int. 2005;15(6):197.

Refining Techniques in Beard and Eyebrow Restoration

10

Anthony Bared

When most think of hair transplantation, the perception is that of restoring hair to the scalp in areas that have suffered hair loss. However, over the last decade, there has been a significant increased demand with patients for facial hair transplantation procedures. Partly as a consequence of social, fashion, and cultural trends, patients are seeking restoration of thinning eyebrows and the transplantation of hair to the beard in ever-increasing numbers. Refinements in techniques in hair transplantation have allowed for the restoration of beard hair and eyebrow hair with very natural appearing results. Pick up any of the latest fashion magazines and you see female models with thick, full eyebrows, or men sporting full beards. Facial hair transplantation is a subspecialty within hair restoration, which while provides many benefits to the hair restoration patient it is also very rewarding to the hair restoration surgeon. Adapting these advanced techniques into a hair restoration practice allows a surgeon to offer their patients these procedures and provides an expanded artistic element to a hair restoration surgeon's practice. In this chapter, hair restoration surgeons will learn how to best select a candidate for facial hair and eyebrow restoration, fine tune the technical and surgical aspects of the procedures, become aware of potential pitfalls, and learn how to best prevent and handle complications of these procedures.

Beard Transplantation

Patient Candidacy and Consultation

Patients for facial hair transplantation typically present with a rather specific idea of how they want their facial hair to appear. Most patients seeking facial hair restoration are men with a genetic paucity of facial hair. Other reasons for patients seeking facial

A. Bared (✉)
South Miami Hospital, Department of Otolaryngology, Miami, FL, USA
e-mail: abared@dranthonybared.com

© Springer Nature Switzerland AG 2020
L. N. Lee (ed.), *Hair Transplant Surgery and Platelet Rich Plasma*,
https://doi.org/10.1007/978-3-030-54648-9_10

Fig. 10.1 Patient with acne scarring presenting for facial hair restoration to help camouflage scars

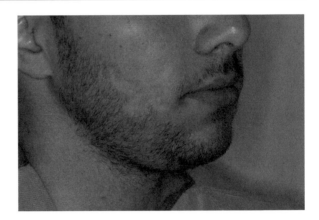

hair restoration are for poorly thought out prior laser hair removal, scarring, burn, or cleft lip repair (Fig. 10.1). Another small group are female-to-male transgender patients seeking a more masculine appearance. It is common for the patient presenting for beard hair restoration to bring with them photos of their "goal" beard shape and density. A patient's goals may vary from increasing the density of an existing beard while maintaining the same shape to transplanting full beards where very few hairs exist. The design and density of the beard may be limited by the quality and quantity of the donor area. Transplantation of full beards requires large amount of grafts, and patients are always made aware of the possibility of undergoing secondary procedures after around 1 year if further density is desired. The hair restoration surgeon needs to guide the patient as to what can be realistically achieved through a procedure. Limitations as to the extent of the height of the cheek beard hair or the coverage of the chin/goatee region are made aware to the patient. Depending on the exact design and density, graft counts can range from 250 to 300 grafts to each sideburn, 400 to 800 grafts to the mustache and goatee, and 300 to 500 grafts per cheek. These numbers can vary based on the preexisting hair, design, and thickness of the donor hair. These grafts, it must be made clear, once transplanted will no longer be available for use in the scalp in the future. if male pattern hair loss is to develop.

It is important for the hair restoration surgeon, starting in beard hair transplantation to have an appreciation for the various levels of complexity certain beard designs present. The novice surgeon should ideally start with smaller cases and transplanting within areas of the beard which pose less of a challenge. The most challenging areas of a beard to create density are those of the central face – mustache, goatee, and the connection of the mustache to the goatee. The cases that pose the greatest challenge are those where the patient has little to no hair in these areas. It is more prudent for the novice surgeon to commence with cases where patients may have existing hair in these areas where the main goal is that of increasing density. It is less challenging to create density in the cheek beard than in the central face. It is particularly very challenging to create density in the region connecting the mustache to the goatee. Patients need to be made aware of these limitations to the creation of density to the mustache and goatee region, so proper expectations are created.

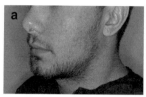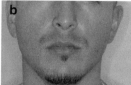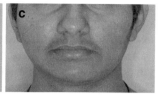

Fig. 10.2 (a–c) Patients with increasing complexity for facial hair restoration. (a) Least challenging presentation of a patient with patchiness to the beard hair. (b) Slightly more challenging presentation of a patient with good density of the mustache but seeking to connect the mustache with the goatee. (c) Most challenging presentation of a patient with little to no facial hair seeking beard transplantation

Donor hair analysis as in any other area of hair restoration is imperative to the preoperative planning. Patients with thick, dark, and very straight donor hair pose the greatest challenge in facial hair restoration. Patients with these donor hair characteristics are more at risk of taking a more unnatural appearance. This author advises starting with smaller-sized cases in patients beard transplantation: patient candidacy and consultation with these donor hair characteristics until one gains the experience needed in facial hair transplantation (Fig. 10.2a–c).

With refinements in FUE, most patients elect to have the procedure performed in this manner so as to avoid a linear scar, allowing them to maintain a short hairstyle [1, 2]. FUE has largely replaced the traditional strip donor extractions for beard transplantation [3]. Regardless of the donor technique used, patients are made aware of the potential limitations of the donor hair quantity and, therefore, "size" and beard transplantation:patient candidacy and consultation density of the beard, which can be achieved through solely one procedure. Scalp hair transplants to the face have a very high regrowth percentage, and if properly performed, patients can achieve a very natural outcome.

Preoperative Planning

There is no ideal facial hair pattern, and there are many differences among different ethnic groups [4]. As mentioned, most patients have a specific idea of the design they wish for their facial hair. On the day of the procedure, the patient is met in the preoperative suite. Using the patient's guidelines, the areas to be transplanted are marked out using a surgical marking pen with the patient in a seated position. The markings are checked for symmetry between the two sides. Measurements are used to help ensure symmetry. Areas where symmetry are most attended to are in the width of each sideburn, the line of curvature connecting the sideburn to the cheek beard, the level at which the cheek beard connects with the mustache, and the width of the connection between the mustache and the goatee. Patients are shown the markings in a mirror, for the two-dimensional perspective provided by a mirror – which is what the patient sees in a mirror – is different than what the surgeon sees in direct three dimension. As previously discussed with the patient during the consultation, limitations may exist as to how high the cheek beard hair may extend, for instance. If then needed, alterations are made according to patient desires.

The one area of caution in patients with thick or dark hair is the area immediately inferior to the lower lip referred to as the "soul patch" area and the chin mound. Particularly in patients with thick and dark hairs, this area is susceptible to bump formation at each graft site. Because of the risk of bump formation, this area is avoided or a few "test" grafts are placed in this area at the time of the initial procedure. If no bumps form after 8 months, then further grafting can be done to this area.

Surgical Procedure

Nearly, all patients seeking facial hair restoration elect to have their procedure via the FUE technique in order to avoid a linear scar. In these cases, the donor area is shaved and patients are placed in a supine position. A handheld drill with the smallest possible drill size avoiding graft transection is used for the extractions. The donor area consists of the occiput only in smaller cases and extends into the parietal scalp for larger cases. Graft extractions are evenly distributed throughout the donor area to avoid areas of focal alopecia. Once the extractions have been completed from the occipital area, the patient is then turned to lie in the supine position. Follicular units utilized are those of one, two, and three hair grafts [5]. In cases of patients with thick and dark donor hairs, the three hair grafts are divided into single and two hair grafts.

Local anesthesia is then applied to the face starting in each sideburn and cheek area. The area around the mouth is not anesthetized at this point, but rather the area around the mouth is typically worked on after the patient has eaten lunch. The recipient sites in the sideburn and cheek area are made first. The smallest possible recipient sites are made using 0.6-, 0.7-, or 0.8-mm slits. The one, two, and (if used) three hair grafts are tested to ensure size compatibility with the recipient sites. In the periphery of the sideburns, one hair graft is used, while two hair grafts can be placed in the central aspect of the sideburn to allow for more density (Fig. 10.3). Counter traction is provided by the nondominant hand and an assistant while making the incisions. The key aesthetic step is to make the incisions at an ultra-acute angle to the skin, with the direction of the incisions determined by either existing surrounding hairs or the fine "peach fuzz" of the face. This being said, the direction of growth is generally downward, but more centrally closer to the mouth/goatee region and can be somewhat anterior (Fig. 10.4). In the cheek area, three hair grafts are sometimes used in the central beard in patients with finer hair to allow for the achievement of greater density without a compromise of naturalness. If further grafts are needed, they are extracted at this time from the parietal scalp. The patient's head is slightly turned, allowing for the simultaneous extraction of grafts from the parietal area and the placement of grafts in the ipsilateral cheek and sideburn.

Fig. 10.3 Figure demonstrates the distribution of follicle graft sizes

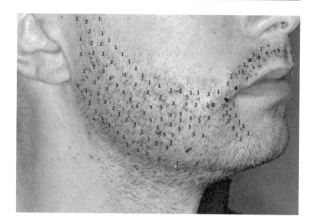

Fig. 10.4 Figure demonstrates the direction of hair growth in most beards

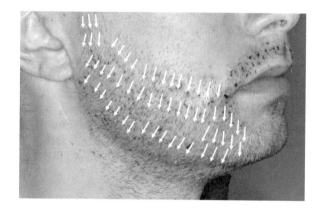

After the patient is given lunch, the area around the mouth is then anesthetized. Infraorbital and mental nerve blocks are used to provide initial anesthesia. The goatee and mustache area anesthesia is then reinforced with field subdermal local anesthesia complemented by epi 1:50,000 to minimize bleeding. Incisions in the goatee and mustache area are then made. On the mustache, hairs will grow slightly laterally and then transition downward along the goatee. As previously mentioned, patients need to be made aware of the difficulty in creating density along the entire mustache, particularly centrally within the "cupid's bow." The creation of density in this area is difficult owing to the undulations created by the upper lip's "cupid's bow" area. It is also important to maintain as acute of an angle as possible in this central area of the upper lip as grafts have a tendency to grow straight outward in nonacute angles. The transition from the mustache to the goatee is an important area for the creation of density, which is usually created by the maximal dense packing of two hair grafts.

The grafts are placed into these recipients using jeweler's forceps. Countertraction splaying the incision sites open with the nondominant hand helps in the placement of the grafts given the laxity of facial skin. The importance of having experienced

Fig. 10.5 Immediate
postoperative results

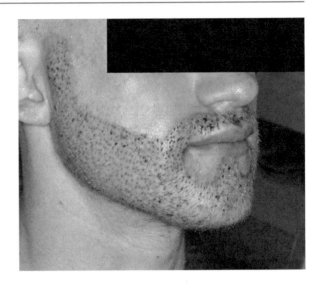

assistants for this process is critical, as they need to understand the "pattern" of graft distribution as created by the surgeon. Toward the conclusion of the case, the patient is given a mirror before all grafts are placed. Given that the immediate results closely replicate the final results, it is helpful for the patient to view their beard in order to assess the design and density of the grafts. This allows for feedback, fine-tuning, and alteration before the conclusion of the case (Fig. 10.5).

Potential Complications and Their Management

Hairs can grow out perpendicularly giving the beard an unnatural appearance. The area of the face where improper angulation poses the greatest challenge is in the mustache particularly in patients with very straight hair. To avoid the improper angulation, it is helpful to use the smallest possible incision at a very acute angle. It is helpful to use a longer blade so as to allow it to lay flat across the skin permitting a sharply acute angle. If needed, the perpendicular hair grafts can be removed via the FUE technique, and the resulting hole is left to heal by secondary intention.

Tiny bumps can form in the soul patch and chin mound areas at the site of the transplanted grafts. The etiology for the formation of these bumps is not known; however, this is mostly seen in patients with thick, dark hairs. Patients of Asian ethnicity, particularly those with dark thick hairs, are the most challenging on whom to avoid complications, both in this bump formation but also in achieving natural-ness due to the difficulty in getting the grafts to look natural particularly in angulation. As mentioned, with patients of Asian descent, the less-experienced surgeon is strongly encouraged to proceed conservatively, with the primary use of all single-hair grafts and smaller number of grafts until proficiency is achieved. As the hair grows in this soul patch and chin mound area, a small bump can form where the hair exits the skin. For this reason, if a patient desires hair in these regions, a small "test" procedure can be performed at the time of the initial procedure. If in 6–8 months, no bumps have been formed, then further hair can be transplanted [6].

Postoperative Management

Patients are told to keep the face dry for the first 5 days after the procedure. This allows for the grafts to set properly, helping assure the maintenance of proper angulation. Topical antibiotic ointment is applied to the donor area. Patients are then to wet the face on the sixth postoperative day with soap and water, starting to remove the dried blood and crusts. Shaving is permitted after 10 days.

Pinkness to the face can be present after the procedure and usually resolves after a few weeks. In patients with very light complexion, this pinkness can persist for longer periods. We have found that the oral antihistamine diphenhydramine taken at night before bedtime can help reduce this pinkness. Hair regrowth usually starts around 4–6 months. The transplanted hair can be treated as any other facial hair and allowed to grow out or shaved. While most patients are satisfied with the initial density from one procedure but a secondary, touch-up procedure can be performed after 1 year to create further density.

Eyebrow Restoration

Patient Candidacy and Consultation

The goal in eyebrow restoration is to restore the desired shape and density, and natural direction and angle of growth of eyebrow hair. The most common presentation in women is the thinning of the eyebrows from over-plucking, aging, or genetic causes. In cases of complete eyebrow absence, types of alopecia (such as alopecia totalis) need to be ruled out before considering transplantation [7]. Men typically lose the lateral aspect of the eyebrows with aging and are seeking overall thicker eyebrows. Female patients who have had prior permanent makeup are advised that this may compromise regrowth in the occasional case. These tattoos can often help guide the design of the eyebrows, but occasionally, they were made asymmetrically and are not aesthetic. The majority of female patients are able to draw their desired eyebrows, which is encouraged, but then often require some fine-tuning by the surgeon to create a nicer look.

The donor hair is almost always the scalp because of its reliable regrowth, although other areas of the body can be used as well, but the regrowth is not as reliable nor is supply oftentimes as readily available. In most cases, scalp donor hair extraction is performed from a small "strip" from the occipital scalp. In some cases, for instance, men who wish to keep a very close haircut, the donor hair is harvested via the FUE technique. The transplanted hairs from the scalp have to be trimmed regularly as they will continue to grow like scalp hair.

Preoperative Planning

Patients are seated in front of a mirror in the preoperative suite. Women generally have a very good idea of the shape they desire for their eyebrows. They are asked to bring in photos of "model" eyebrows to help guide their design. After preoperative photos are obtained, the patients are offered an eyeliner pen and are given the time to draw in their desired eyebrow shape if they so desire. The patient's active involvement in the design of their eyebrows is important, whether by demonstrating model photos or drawing in their desired shape. After they are given some time to design their eyebrows, final markings and refinements are made with a semi-permanent fine marker. Measurements are taken for symmetry. Men seeking eyebrow restoration typically are seeking to fill in areas within the eyebrows which are lacking density. The male eyebrow is designed with less of an arch and as an extension of the existing eyebrow. Photos are obtained after the final markings have been made.

The eyebrow can be divided into three areas: head (innermost 5–8 mm), body (central 2.5–3.5 cm), and tail (outer 2–2.5 cm). In women, the point at which the tail and body meet forming the arch is usually located at or just lateral to the lateral limbus of the eye. For a more dramatic look, this arch can be as far lateral to the lateral canthal region. However, it can vary in position and roundedness. In men, the arch of the brow is not so much as a peek but rather a widening of the eyebrow along the area correlating to the lateral limbus (Fig. 10.6).

Procedural Approach

If a "strip" harvesting technique is to be utilized, the patient remains in the upright, seated position for the excision. The "strip" is typically harvested using a trichophytic incision from the occipital scalp and, depending on the number of grafts needed, varies in length and width from about 3–6 cm and 10–15 mm, respectively. If the FUE technique is used, the patient is placed in the prone position for donor harvesting. Given the smaller number of grafts needed, shaving of the entire donor

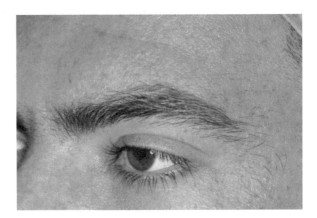

Fig. 10.6 Typical pattern of male eyebrow

area is avoided. Small "tunnels" can be made in various locations throughout the occipital and parietal areas with the surrounding hair kept long to avoid the donor area from becoming visible.

Once the donor hairs have been harvested, the patient is then positioned in a supine/"beach chair" position for incision-site placement. Highly experienced technicians perform the dissection of the harvested donor hairs under the microscope under the supervision of the surgeon. Naturally occurring 1 and 2 hair follicular units are dissected, although in some cases, 3 hair follicular units will be used to achieve maximal density without compromising naturalness. When follicular units greater than one are used, they are analyzed under the microscope to ensure that the hairs are exiting from the skin in parallel direction. It is important to note that the direction of hair growth is not divergent as it helps to ensure that the subsequent grafts are placed in such a manner that the hair is at the most acute angle to the skin.

The eyebrows are anesthetized, and 1:50,000 epi is injected for hemostasis. Recipient sites are created by the surgeon using the smallest blade size appropriate for the grafts, most commonly 0.5 mm, but sometimes 0.6 mm for the occasional larger two hair grafts and even three hair grafts. Recipient sites are first made along the boundaries of the eyebrow along the preoperative markings as these markings can be lost with the subsequent bleeding and wiping of the blood from the recipient sites. Paying attention to the proper direction of growth is critical. Within the head of the eyebrow, hair usually grows in a more vertical/superior direction. Moving from the more inferior to the more superior aspect of the head of the brow, the hairs quickly change direction to grow in a more horizontal then inferior/downward direction particularly along the superior border. Moving laterally, the hairs along the superior border are oriented in an inferior/downward direction, while the hairs along the inferior border are oriented in a superior/upward direction, creating a herringboned pattern. This cross-hatching continues throughout the body of the eyebrow until the tail portion, where the hairs then are primarily oriented horizontally (Fig. 10.7). Incisions are made as flat (acute an angle) as possible to the skin (Fig. 10.8). Once all the recipient sites are made bilaterally, the grafts are then inserted. Care is taken to orient the hairs so that the direction of growth (i.e., the curl) of the hair is in an acute angle with the skin. We like to place as many two hair grafts as possible, except along the innermost head and lateralmost tail portion where one hair graft is used. If three hair grafts are deemed appropriate, they are

Fig. 10.7 Figure demonstrating the direction of eyebrow hair growth and the distribution of graft size within the eyebrow

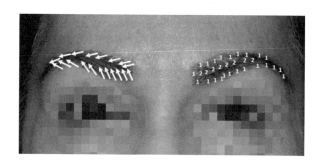

Fig. 10.8 Incisions are
made with the smallest
possible blade size to
accommodate the grafts at
a very acute angle to
the skin

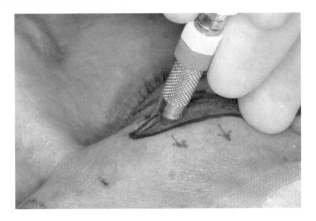

placed in the central aspect of the body portion, to achieve maximal density. It is critical to make just about all of the recipient sites before any planting is to be done, then after all these recipient sites are filled with grafts, the patient is asked to sit up and the eyebrows are inspected, and then small adjustments can be made with the placement of more grafts. Then, the patient can then view the eyebrows to obtain his/her feedback regarding the desired shape.

Potential Complications and Their Management

The most common complications related to eyebrow hair restorations are asymmetry, less than anticipate hair regrowth, and poor hair angulation. It is important when marking the eyebrows that symmetry is checked and rechecked. It is also helpful to view the immediate photo once the markings have been made. The viewing of the photos helps to provide a "third" eye and different perspective often revealing asymmetries which may not have been immediately apparent. As aforementioned, recipient sites are first made along these markings along the boundaries of the eyebrow before they can be rubbed off and lost. The local anesthesia and the swelling can create asymmetries during the procedure, making one eyebrow appear higher than the other and thus creating artifactual asymmetric appearances that are more difficult to correct at the end of the procedure. To limit this phenomenon, it is best to place the local anesthetic in the very beginning of the case and to have the patient sit up to check for symmetry before adding more local anesthetic during the procedure.

Another potential complication is that related to poor density. This is most likely due to lower than expected percentage of regrowth. Despite the best efforts to keep the grafts moist as well as atraumatic placement of the grafts, at times, in certain cases, 20–25% of the hair may fail to regrow. To minimize poor regrowth rates, the grafts are kept "chubby" with a small cuff of surrounding protective fat, and the most experienced assistants perform the insertion of the grafts. Patients are advised that this is not necessarily a complication but rather something that simply sometimes occurs, and thus, a second smaller procedure can be performed after 10 months or more to achieve greater density.

   Lastly, poor hair growth angulation can occur in the occasional case despite the best efforts in acute recipient-site angulation and hair placement. This is likely due to the effects of healing and subtle wound contracture. It is most commonly seen in patients with very straight hair not allowing for the harvesting of the natural curl to assure flat growth of hairs. To best help prevent this, a very acute angle is taken with the skin when making recipient sites and rotating the hair upon insertion so that the natural curl of the hair is aimed downward. It is also best not to trim the hair in the donor area – if by strip – in order to better visualize the hair curl.

Postprocedure Care

Patients are instructed to keep the eyebrows dry for the first 5 days. If "strip" harvesting was performed, sutures are removed around 10 days postoperatively or the dissolvable sutures are expected to be gone by 4 weeks. Antibiotics and pain medications are given for the first several days. Patients are allowed to use makeup in the eyebrow area after all the crusts have fallen out at typically 5 days.

   Eyebrows will start to regrow around 4–6 months after transplant and will continue to fill in for a full year, gradually increasing density. A variety of products can be used to train any misdirected hairs. The hair must be trimmed to the patient's desired length. If a patient so desires, second smaller procedures to increase density are performed 10 months or later.

References

1. Rassman WR, Berstein RM, McClellan R, et al. Follicular unit extraction: minimally invasive surgery for hair transplantation. Dermatol Surg. 2002;28:720–8.
2. Harris J. Conventional FUE in hair transplantation. In: Unger W, Shapiro R, Unger R, editors. Hair transplantation. 5th ed; 2001. p. 291–6.
3. Unger W, Shapiro R, Unger R, et al. Donor area harvesting. In: Hair transplantation. 5th ed. New York: Informa Healthcare; 2011. p. 247–90.
4. Gandelman M, Epstein JS. Reconstruction of the sideburn, moustache, and beard. Facial Plast Surg Clin North Am. 2004;12:253–61.
5. Unger WP. On: follicular transplantation by Bernstein and Rassman. Dermatol Surg. 1997;23(9):801–5. doi: 10.1111/j.1524-4725.1997.tb00421.x. PMID: 9340102.
6. Epstein JS. Hair restoration to eyebrows, beard, sideburns, and eyelashes. Facial Plast Surg Clin North Am. 2013;21:457–67.
7. Tosti A, Piraccini BM. Diagnosis and treatment of hair disorders: an evidence based atlas. New York: Informa Healthcare; 2005.

Platelet-Rich Plasma for Hair Restoration

11

Natalie Justicz, Jenny X. Chen, and Linda N. Lee

Introduction

Hair loss is treated with a wide range of clinical therapies including low-level laser light therapy as well as two FDA-approved medications: topical minoxidil and oral finasteride. Surgical options include follicular unit transplant (FUT) and follicular unit extraction (FUE) techniques, which are outpatient procedures with excellent outcomes. In addition to these existing medical and surgical options, platelet-rich plasma (PRP) is a relatively new, minimally invasive, office-based procedure used to treat hair loss, typically secondary to androgenic alopecia (AGA). PRP consists of growth factors extracted from autologous blood obtained by venipuncture. This concentrated mix of growth factors is injected into areas of hair loss, stimulating hair regrowth.

Platelet-rich plasma (PRP), alternatively called platelet-rich growth factors or platelet concentrate, was first described in the field of hematology in the 1970s [1]. Hematologists coined the term PRP to describe a high-platelet product used for the treatment of thrombocytopenia. Within the fields of orthopedics and sports medicine, PRP has been touted for its ability to stimulate soft tissue and joint healing due to its high concentration of growth factors. Since the 1990s, PRP has been used to promote wound healing across a number of medical fields including

N. Justicz · J. X. Chen
Massachusetts Eye and Ear, Department of Otolaryngology-Head and Neck Surgery, Harvard Medical School, Boston, MA, USA

L. N. Lee (✉)
Facial Plastic and Reconstructive Surgery, Assistant Professor, Harvard Medical School, Massachusetts Eye and Ear, Associate Chief of Plastic Surgery, Harvard Vanguard Medical Associates, Boston, MA, USA
e-mail: Linda_Lee@meei.harvard.edu

© Springer Nature Switzerland AG 2020
L. N. Lee (ed.), *Hair Transplant Surgery and Platelet Rich Plasma*,
https://doi.org/10.1007/978-3-030-54648-9_11

ophthalmology, OMFS, cardiac surgery, gynecology, and urology [2, 3]. More recently, the growth factor concentrate has become of interest to facial plastic surgeons, dermatologists, and those interested in its possible aesthetic applications and additional off-label uses.

According to the FDA, blood products like PRP fall under regulations set forth by the Center for Biologics Evaluation and Research (CBER) which regulates human cells, tissues, and cellular and tissue-based products [4]. Certain products including PRP are exempt and therefore do not follow the FDA's traditional regulatory pathway that necessitate animal studies and clinical trials [4]. Nearly all preparation systems for PRP were designed to generate platelet concentrate to be mixed with bone graft material for orthopedic applications [4]. Despite this, PRP is often used for a range of off-label applications. Uses for PRP in the field of facial plastic and reconstructive surgery include soft tissue augmentation [5], skin rejuvenation [6, 7], and wound healing [8, 9], as well as hair restoration.

A recent review by Sand et al. examined the early body of evidence for PRP in aesthetic surgery, including hair loss and facial rejuvenation [10]. Sand et al. concluded that PRP has been considered a promising new therapy for androgenic alopecia (AGA). One of the earliest articles on this application was published in 2006 by Uebel et al. who described a 15% greater hair yield in follicular unit density in areas pre-treated with PRP as compared to controls [11]. This inspired interest and fueled the development of PRP technology for hair restoration and its clinical adoption. A more recent systematic review paper by Chen et al. examined PRP for hair restoration specifically in patients with AGA [12]. Patient demographics, frequency of treatment, hair count, and hair density following PRP therapy were analyzed with promising results [12]. The hair restoration community is investing considerable resources in the development of PRP therapies. The following is a summary of current knowledge of PRP for hair restoration to date, with the caveat that this field is rapidly evolving.

Platelet-Rich Plasma Mechanism of Action

Many growth factors have been identified in PRP including platelet-derived growth factor, transforming growth factor-β, vascular endothelial growth factor, epidermal growth factor, and insulin-like growth factor (Table 11.1). These factors are present in much higher concentrations (by five to eight times) in PRP than in whole blood and PRP has been shown to induce the proliferation of dermal papilla cells by upregulating FGF-7, beta-catenin, and ERK/Akt signaling through these factors [17]. Though these factors are upregulated in PRP, the precise biological pathways by which PRP promotes hair restoration remain largely unknown. One proposed mechanism is that growth factors released from platelets act in the bulge area of hair follicles where stem cells are found, stimulating the development of new follicles and promoting neovascularization [11, 18].

Table 11.1 Main functions of the growth factors present to platelet-rich plasma

Growth factors	Main functions
PDGF [13]	Increases hair growth
	Vascularization
	Angiogenesis stimulators
TGF-β [14]	Inhibits hair growth in vitro
	Hair-cell proliferation and regeneration
VEGF [15]	Expressed in DP cells in the anagen phase
	Probably regulates perifollicular angiogenesis
	Increases perifollicular vessel size during the anagen growth phase
EG F [14, 43]	Angiogenesis stimulator
	Hair-cell proliferation and regeneration
HGF [16]	Angiogenesis stimulator
FGF [14, 43–45]	Increases hair growth by inducing the anagen phase of HF
	Promotes DP cell proliferation
	Increases the HF size in mice
	Angiogenesis stimulators
IGF-1 [6, 13, 46]	Increases hair growth
	Maintaines HF growth in vitro
	Angiogenesis stimulator

PDGF platelet-derived growth factor, *TGF* transforming growth factor, *VEGF* vascular endothelial growth factor, *DP* dermal papilla, *EGF* epidermal growth factor, *HGF* hepatocyte growth factor, *FGF* fibroblast growth factor, *IGF-1* insulin-like growth factor 1, *HF* human follicle(s)

Pre-procedure Considerations and Testing

Patients seeking PRP for hair restoration are commonly those who have not experienced success with finasteride or minoxidil for the treatment of androgenic alopecia (AGA). AGA is a disease of progressive hair loss mediated by systemic androgens and other genetic factors. It is the most common type of hair loss for patients of both genders. AGA affects greater than 73% of men and greater than 57% of women by the age of 80 [19, 20]. As much as 58% of the male population between 30 and 50 years of age has AGA [21]. Many patients present to PCPs, dermatologists, plastics surgeons, and otolaryngologists for counseling regarding hair restoration therapies. As in any encounter leading to a prescription medication or procedural treatment, a full history and physical exam are imperative.

The diagnosis of AGA must be established based on detailed medical history, medication history, and clinical examination. Laboratory tests should be performed to exclude other causes of hair loss such as anemia, malnutrition, and thyroid dysfunction. This laboratory work often includes a complete blood cell count including a measurement of serum levels of iron, serum ferritin, total iron-binding capacity, and folic acid. Thyroid function laboratory tests include T3, T4, thyroid stimulating hormone, and antithyroid peroxidase. Other endocrine tests may include a measure of testosterone and other hormones. Autoimmune markers such as ANA may also be drawn. Some physicians confirm diagnosis of AGA with scalp biopsy.

After other medical causes of hair loss have been excluded, the patient and physician can consider the use of medications and treatments. Many patients with AGA start by trying FDA-approved medications. If minoxidil and/or finasteride do not provide significant improvement, patients become more willing to investigate more invasive procedures.

PRP does not take the place of hair transplant via FUT or FUE. Rather, it should be considered in patients who may wish to stabilize hair loss or who are not ready to move forward with transplant, acting as a stand-alone procedure to maintain or improve hair density and hair count. It can also be considered as an adjuvant to hair transplant.

Some additional contraindications exist when determining whether a patient is safe for PRP therapy. Patients with coagulopathies are generally not considered good candidates for PRP therapy and have largely been excluded from trials based on concern for periprocedural bleeding. Patients on anticoagulation or anti-platelet medications (such a clopidigrel or aspirin) should also be considered carefully, as they may also be at higher risk for bleeding. Moreover, as the mechanism of PRP may be related to the concentration and activity of platelets and platelet-derived factors, patients on anti-platelet medications were excluded from most studies to date and therefore it is unclear whether they will see the same benefits. Reassuringly, a study within the cardiac surgery literature shows no statistical evidence of decreased growth factors delivered to the surgical wound site in the presence of aspirin and/or clopidigrel use [22], but it is unclear whether this is generalizable to hair restoration treatments with PRP.

PRP Preparation

PRP is prepared from a patient's autologous blood sample. An 18–30-cc venous blood draw yields 3–5 cc of PRP depending on the harvesting technique or preparation kit. There are many methods of creating PRP, but most have some steps in common. Blood is collected in tubes lined with anticoagulant, which are immediately centrifuged to separate the blood into three layers: red blood cells (RBCs) are at the bottom, acellular plasma (PPP, platelet-poor plasma) is in the supernatant, and a buffy coat layer appears in the middle where platelets and leukocytes are concentrated in platelet-rich plasma (Fig. 11.1) [3]. The subsequent steps vary between protocols as to which layers are harvested, but there is a general attempt to discard much of both the RBC layer and the PPP to collect only the material surrounding the buffy coat. After platelet-poor fluid has been discarded, the resultant platelet concentrate is applied to the surgical site. The time for platelet concentrate preparation can typically be completed in less than 1 hour.

Fig. 11.1 Blood is separated into three layers after centrifugation: erythrocytes, platelet-poor plasma (PPP), and platelet-rich plasma (PRP). PPP is typically discarded and the PRP is drawn and prepared for injection

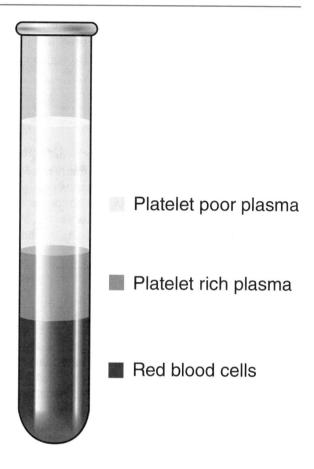

Platelet poor plasma

Platelet rich plasma

Red blood cells

PRP Administration

PRP is injected into areas of hair loss using a small-gauge needle such as a 30-gauge needle or an insulin syringe. While PRP has also been used in the literature as topical sprays [23, 24], the vast majority of described techniques involve injections of small aliquots of PRP into the subcutaneous layer of the scalp. A local anesthetic such as lidocaine can be used, although the majority of described techniques in the literature do not describe the use of numbing agent. Lidocaine is not reported to disrupt hair growth, although this has not been well studied. Alternatively, topical analgesia can also be applied as well as ice for vasoconstriction. In addition, the Zimmer cooler from a laser can be used during the injection for comfort.

Treatment areas can include the frontal, parietal, and occipital scalp. Typically, activated PRP is used, created by treating PRP with calcium chloride to activate platelets. Chen et al. found that the majority of studies used more than one treatment of PRP per patient, with most offering between 3 and 6 treatments with 1 month between injections [12]. Patients should therefore be counseled to expect multiple rounds of treatment to maximize results.

Post-procedure Considerations

Few studies have noted any complications from PRP treatment. Some report temporary pain during injections [24, 25] and transient edema/erythema at the injection site [18, 26]. No allergic reactions, hematomas, or infections have been documented.

Patients can be counseled that there is no contraindication to showering or exercising following treatment. No antibiotic is needed. Most patients are able to return to work the next day. No significant or lasting swelling is anticipated.

PRP Outcomes

Multiple retrospective studies, prospective trials, and systematic reviews suggest that PRP may be a promising new treatment for AGA. However, additional research is still needed to optimize the use of PRP for hair restoration.

The best use of PRP in terms of preparation, activation, and treatment regimens is unknown. Dohan Ehrenfest et al. describe a classification system of platelet concentrates based on preparatory process and leukocyte and fibrin content: P-PRP (pure platelet-rich plasma), L-PRP (leukocyte- and platelet-rich plasma), P-PRF (pure platelet-rich fibrin), and L-PRF (leukocyte and platelet-rich fibrin) [3]. The majority of published studies use to date an L-PRP derivate [12].

In the largest systematic review by Chen et al., 21 of 24 studies examining the effect of PRP on hair restoration reported positive outcomes (88%), both subjective and objective [12]. Thirteen studies (54%) reported statistically significant improvement in at least one outcome that could be measured objectively. Hair counts or hair densities were described by 16 studies [14, 15, 18, 25–36] and of these, 12 found statistically significant improvements in this outcome. Among studies with the highest level of evidence, 6 of 8 (75%) of RCTs reported positive treatment outcomes. Three studies did not report positive findings after PRP administration including two RCTs [16, 32], but these continued to report high patient satisfaction treatment results.

Future research should study the use of PRP in combination with minoxidil and finasteride. Most studies have excluded patients taking topical or oral medication within a certain time period of study initiation (e.g., 60 days or 12 months) so as to avoid confounding results. However, for many patients, it could make sense to try topical and oral medications in conjunction with PRP to maximize hair restoration potential. These patients would still be candidates for FUT and FUE hair transplant technology, which can be completed in conjunction with PRP therapy.

As patients with AGA can be affected at a young age, longer follow-up of patients is required to determine whether this treatment has long-lasting effects or whether repeated injections could be considered. In the literature, the shortest follow-up time for studies was 6 weeks and the longest was 1 year [12]. Additionally, only 28% of patients in the systematic review performed by Chen et al. were female; there remains limited information on potential gender differences in the effect of PRP [12].

The preponderance of evidence related to PRP and hair restoration is positive. It is becoming a more common procedure in hair restoration practices. Clinicians should familiarize themselves with the expanding repertoire of hair restoration treatments available to patients to provide individualized hair loss therapy.

Conclusions

PRP is a promising treatment for hair restoration in patients with androgenic alopecia. Created from a platelet concentrate from an autologous blood draw, PRP is a safe therapeutic option for patients with hair loss. It can be used alone or in conjunction with topical and oral therapies. PRP may also be administered before FUT or FUE.

Most studies of hair restoration with PRP report positive outcomes. Further research to optimize PRP preparation/administration procedures and identify patient populations that benefit most from this treatment is needed, in addition to long-term follow-up of objective hair loss outcomes. PRP appears to be a safe technology with excellent potential for promoting hair restoration.

References

1. Matras H. Effect of various fibrin preparations on reimplantations in the rat skin. Osterr Z Stomatol. 1970;67(9):338–59. German. PubMed PMID: 4917644.
2. Marx RE, Carlson ER, Eichstaedt RM, Schimmele SR, Strauss JE, Georgeff KR. Platelet-rich plasma: growth factor enhancement for bone grafts. Oral Surg Oral Med Oral Pathol Oral Radiol Endod. 1998;85:638–46.
3. Dohan Ehrenfest DM, Rasmusson L, Albrektsson T. Classification of platelet concentrates: from pure platelet-rich plasma (P-PRP) to leucocyte- and platelet-rich fibrin (L-PRF). Trends Biotechnol. 2009;27(3):158–67. https://doi.org/10.1016/j.tibtech.2008.11.009.
4. Beitzel K, Allen D, Apostolakos J, et al. US definitions, current use, and FDA stance on use of platelet-rich plasma in sports medicine. J Knee Surg. 2015;28(1):29–34. https://doi.org/10.105 5/s-0034-1390030.
5. Ulusal BG. Platelet-rich plasma and hyaluronic acid - an efficient biostimulation method for face rejuvenation. J Cosmet Dermatol. 2017;16(1):112–9. https://doi.org/10.1111/jocd.12271.
6. Asif M, Kanodia S, Singh K. Combined autologous platelet-rich plasma with microneedling verses microneedling with distilled water in the treatment of atrophic acne scars: a concurrent split-face study. J Cosmet Dermatol. 2016;15(4):434–43. https://doi.org/10.1111/jocd.12207.
7. Shin M-K, Lee J-H, Lee S-J, Kim N-I. Platelet-rich plasma combined with fractional laser therapy for skin rejuvenation. Dermatol Surg. 2012;38(4):623–30. https://doi.org/10.1111/j.1524-4725.2011.02280.x.

8. Kang J-S, Zheng Z, Choi MJ, Lee S-H, Kim D-Y, Cho SB. The effect of CD34+ cell-containing autologous platelet-rich plasma injection on pattern hair loss: a preliminary study. J Eur Acad Dermatol Venereol. 2014;28(1):72–9. https://doi.org/10.1111/jdv.12062.

9. Sclafani AP, Azzi J. Platelet preparations for use in facial rejuvenation and wound healing: a critical review of current literature. Aesthet Plast Surg. 2015;39(4):495–505. https://doi.org/10.1007/s00266-015-0504-x.

10. Sand JP, Nabili V, Kochhar A, Rawnsley J, Keller G. Platelet-rich plasma for the aesthetic surgeon. Facial Plast Surg. 2017;33(04):437–43.

11. Uebel CO, da Silva JB, Cantarelli D, Martins P. The role of platelet plasma growth factors in male pattern baldness surgery. Plast Reconstr Surg. 2006;118(6):1458–66.

12. Chen JX, Justicz N, Lee LN. Platelet-rich plasma for the treatment of androgenic alopecia: a systematic review. Facial Plastic Surg. 2018;34:631.

13. Marwah M, Godse K, Patil S, Nadkarni N. Is there sufficient research data to use platelet-rich plasma in dermatology? Int J Trichol. 2014;6(1):35–6. https://doi.org/10.4103/0974-7753.136763.

14. Takikawa M, Nakamura S, Nakamura S, et al. Enhanced effect of platelet-rich plasma containing a new carrier on hair growth. Dermatol Surg. 2011;37(12):1721–9. https://doi.org/10.1111/j.1524-4725.2011.02123.x.

15. Sclafani AP. Platelet-rich fibrin matrix (PRFM) for androgenetic alopecia. Facial Plast Surg. 2014;30(2):219–24. https://doi.org/10.1055/s-0034-1371896.

16. Mapar MA, Shahriari S, Haghighizadeh MH. Efficacy of platelet-rich plasma in the treatment of androgenetic (male-patterned) alopecia: a pilot randomized controlled trial. J Cosmet Laser Ther. 2016;18(8):452–5. https://doi.org/10.1080/14764172.2016.1225963.

17. Gupta AK, Carviel J. A mechanistic model of platelet-rich plasma treatment for androgenetic alopecia. Dermatol Surg. 2016;42(12):1335–9. https://doi.org/10.1097/DSS.0000000000000901.

18. Khatu SS, More YE, Gokhale NR, Chavhan DC, Bendsure N. Platelet-rich plasma in androgenic alopecia: myth or an effective tool. J Cutan Aesthetic Surg. 2014;7(2):107–10. https://doi.org/10.4103/0974-2077.138352.

19. Hamilton JB. Patterned loss of hair in man: types and incidence. Ann N Y Acad Sci. 1951;53(3):708–28. https://doi.org/10.1111/j.1749-6632.1951.tb31971.x.

20. Gan DCC, Sinclair RD. Prevalence of male and female pattern hair loss in Maryborough. J Investig Dermatol Symp Proc. 2005;10(3):184–9. https://doi.org/10.1111/j.1087-0024.2005.10102.x.

21. Krupa Shankar D, Chakravarthi M, Shilpakar R. Male androgenetic alopecia: population-based study in 1,005 subjects. Int J Trichol. 2009;1(2):131–3. https://doi.org/10.4103/0974-7753.58556.

22. Smith CW, Binford RS, Holt DW, Webb DP. Quality assessment of platelet rich plasma during anti-platelet therapy. Perfusion. 2007;22(1):41–50.

23. James R, Chetry R, Subramanian V, et al. Platelet-rich plasma growth factor concentrated spray (Keratogrow®) as a potential treatment for androgenic alopecia. J Stem Cells. 2016;11(4):183–9.

24. Farid CI, Abdelmaksoud RA. Platelet-rich plasma microneedling versus 5% topical minoxidil in the treatment of patterned hair loss. J Egypt Women's Dermatol Soc. 2016;13(1):29. https://doi.org/10.1097/01.EWX.0000472824.29209.a8.

25. Tawfik AA, Osman MAR. The effect of autologous activated platelet-rich plasma injection on female pattern hair loss: a randomized placebo-controlled study. J Cosmet Dermatol. 2017;17:47. https://doi.org/10.1111/jocd.12357.

26. Anitua E, Pino A, Martinez N, Orive G, Berridi D. The effect of plasma rich in growth factors on pattern hair loss: a pilot study. Dermatol Surg. 2017;43(5):658–70. https://doi.org/10.1097/DSS.0000000000001049.

27. Kachhawa D, Vats G, Sonare D, Rao P, Khuraiya S, Kataiya R. A spilt head study of efficacy of placebo versus platelet-rich plasma injections in the treatment of androgenic alopecia. J Cutan Aesthet Surg. 2017;10(2):86–9. https://doi.org/10.4103/JCAS.JCAS_50_16.
28. Rodrigues BL, Montalvão SADL, Annichinno-Bizzacchi J, et al. The therapeutic response of platelet rich plasma (PRP) for androgenetic alopecia showed no correlation with growth factors and platelet number. Blood. 2016;128(22):2637.
29. Borhan R, Gasnier C, Reygagne P. Autologous platelet rich plasma as a treatment of male androgenetic alopecia: study of 14 cases. J Clin Exp Dermatol Res. 2015;6(4):4. https://doi.org/10.4172/2155-9554.10000292.
30. Gkini M-A, Kouskoukis A-E, Tripsianis G, Rigopoulos D, Kouskoukis K. Study of platelet-rich plasma injections in the treatment of androgenetic alopecia through an one-year period. J Cutan Aesthet Surg. 2014;7(4):213–9. https://doi.org/10.4103/0974-2077.150743.
31. Gentile P, Cole JP, Cole MA, et al. Evaluation of not-activated and activated PRP in hair loss treatment: role of growth factor and cytokine concentrations obtained by different collection systems. Int J Mol Sci. 2017;18(2):408. https://doi.org/10.3390/ijms18020408.
32. Puig CJ, Reese R, Peters M. Double-blind, placebo-controlled pilot study on the use of platelet-rich plasma in women with female androgenetic alopecia. Dermatol Surg. 2016;42(11):1243–7. https://doi.org/10.1097/DSS.0000000000000883.
33. Gentile P, Garcovich S, Bielli A, Scioli MG, Orlandi A, Cervelli V. The effect of platelet-rich plasma in hair regrowth: a randomized placebo-controlled trial. Stem Cells Transl Med. 2015;4(11):1317–23. https://doi.org/10.5966/sctm.2015-0107.
34. Alves R, Grimalt R. Randomized placebo-controlled, double-blind, half-head study to assess the efficacy of platelet-rich plasma on the treatment of androgenetic alopecia. Dermatol Surg. 2016;42(4):491–7. https://doi.org/10.1097/DSS.0000000000000665.
35. Cervelli V, Garcovich S, Bielli A, et al. The effect of autologous activated platelet rich plasma (AA-PRP) injection on pattern hair loss: clinical and histomorphometric evaluation. Biomed Res Int. 2014;2014:760709. https://doi.org/10.1155/2014/760709.
36. Kang R, Nimmons GL, Drennan W, et al. Development and validation of the University of Washington Clinical Assessment of Music Perception test. Ear Hear. 2009;30(4):411–8. https://doi.org/10.1097/AUD.0b013e3181a61bc0.

Photography for Evaluating Patients with Hair Loss

12

Dylan Russell and Prabhat K. Bhama

Introduction

Physicians are continuously required by our peers, patients, payers, and the government to provide proof that our interventions are beneficial to the patient, and to measure the quality of our care. These data are in turn used by payers for justifying reimbursement and by patients for selecting a provider. In facial plastic and reconstructive surgery, demonstrating benefit and measuring quality are challenging because of the constructs available to measure our outcomes. Whereas many other medical disciplines can rely on objective measurements to assess the efficacy of their interventions, we are often forced to rely on more subjective concepts such as attractiveness and happiness. As a result, facial plastic surgeons have recently made a concerted effort to develop more objective outcome assessments. Many of these outcomes are direct measurements made from photographs taken of patients in the perioperative period [3] or social perceptions based on a photograph [2].

Ideally, when developing outcome measurements based upon the still photograph medium, strict imaging standards should exist to prevent variation in the development of new outcome measures as a result of inconsistencies in the medium. Non-standardized photography is associated with dramatic variations in reporting the subjective appearance of facial characteristics [5]. Unfortunately, imaging standards are not always available for facial plastic surgery and hair restoration surgery. Because of the recent significant advances in digital camera technology, many photographic concepts are now outdated and need to be revisited. Additionally, as cameras have become more complex, standardizing photography has become more

D. Russell
General Surgery Resident, Tripler Army Medical Center, Honolulu, HI, USA

P. K. Bhama (✉)
University of Hawaii John A. Burns School of Medicine, University of Washington School of Medicine, Seattle, WA, USA

challenging for the surgeon, who often does not have time to read an instruction manual and understand the intricacies of the digital camera, which are not intuitive.

In this chapter, we will review basic concepts in photography. After understanding the concepts covered herein, the reader should be comfortable with several tasks, including using the camera in manual modes, changing depth of field, using available light to achieve proper exposure, and using external lighting sources. We will also discuss previously proposed standardized views for photographing patients with hair loss.

Important Considerations for Medical Photography

Medical photography has several purposes. Perhaps the most important are medico-legal documentation and outcome assessment. As such, it is absolutely crucial to eliminate confounding variables in our photography. In other words, any changes between the pre- and post-intervention photo should be a direct result of the medical or surgical intervention that was performed. Thus, the photographer should ensure consistency in several variables when taking pictures, including exposure, focal length, depth of field, white balance, and lighting. Ideally, the patient would also wear the same clothing and makeup (or no makeup) between the pre- and postoperative photo, but this can be practically challenging. For hair photography, the use of hair products should be avoided, or at least be consistent between photo sessions (Box 12.1). Additionally, several standardized views have been proposed for assessment of patients with alopecia (Box 12.2).

Because it is crucial for the photographer to maintain consistency between photo sessions, understanding the parameters that influence the variables discussed above (exposure, depth of field, etc.), is helpful. Simply placing the camera in "automatic

---

Box 12.1 Important aspects of a photograph that must remain constant pre- and post-intervention

Critical
1. Exposure
2. Focal length
3. Depth of field
4. White balance
5. Lighting

Ideal
1. Clothing
2. Makeup
3. Hair products

Box 12.2 Standard views for patients with alopecia

Anterior hairline
1. Nasal tip in line with inferior earlobe
2. Inferior brow in line with inferior earlobe
3. Nasal tip in line with pogonion

Vertex
1. Subnasale with superior-most aspect of helix
2. Left lateral
3. Left oblique
4. Posterior
5. Right oblique
6. Right lateral views

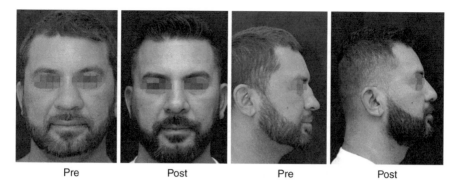

| Pre | Post | Pre | Post |

Fig. 12.1 Change in exposure between photographs results in distraction from the aspect of interest

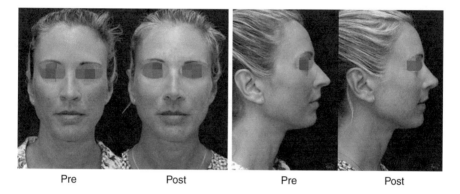

| Pre | Post | Pre | Post |

Fig. 12.2 Photographs with consistent parameters permit assessment of changes resulting from surgical intervention

mode" will surrender this control to the camera's software, allowing it to make its own adjustments. This will introduce variability into your photography, distracting from the variables of interest (e.g., nasal appearance, hairline, etc.) (Fig. 12.1). The camera on your smart phone routinely adjusts its internal parameters to achieve what it feels is the optimal photograph for the situation based on the amount of light available in the image. As a result, photos taken under the automatic mode may be ideally exposed for the particular situation, but are not suitable for medical photography because of the lack in consistency between shots. Therefore, to maintain consistency, the photographer must control the environment in which the images are taken, as well as the parameters in the camera (Fig. 12.2).

Types of Cameras

There are several basic types of cameras available today. In general, one can think of cameras belonging to one of two groups: digital and standard film cameras. Film cameras certainly have their advantages including high dynamic range, excellent resolution, and their independence from requiring power or batteries. Nonetheless, for the medical professional, these subtle (and debatable) advantages are outweighed by the benefits of the digital camera. Digital cameras in the long term can be much more cost effective, since film processing fees are not required. Storage of film and retrieval of images of interest can be cumbersome, whereas with digital images, storage and retrieval are straightforward and have powerful advantages. Perhaps the most crucial advantage of the digital camera is the ability to view the image immediately, permitting the photographer to immediately retake the shot if the desired result was not obtained. Therefore, we will focus on digital cameras in this text.

Rather than using film as the medium for recording light data, the digital camera uses a memory card, (SD, XQD, or CF, etc.). Digital cameras can be grouped into several different classes. These include fixed lens cameras, and interchangeable lens cameras. Fixed lens cameras are also often known as "point-and-shoot/compact" (compact) cameras, or smart phone cameras. Interchangeable lens cameras include digital single-lens reflex and mirrorless.

Fixed Lens ("Point-and-Shoot" or "Compact")

Fixed lens/point-and-shoot cameras (denoted "compact" from this point on) are typically more inexpensive than their other counterparts, but are often more limited in their abilities. Their advantages are primarily physical in nature, as they are small and lightweight. They are also typically geared toward the amateur photographer, and as such are convenient to use in the more automatic modes, but do not provide the same level of manual control as interchangeable lens cameras. The smart phone camera has become quite advanced now, and as such, many individuals have chosen to not carry a compact camera and rely only on their smart phone camera, which is an excellent tool for taking basic photographs.

Many of these cameras also include a built-in flash unit, which I find to be of little use. The built-in flash is handy in certain situations, but generally will flatten out photos by filling in shadows, and overexpose a subject's face. Additionally, since light travels in a straight line, and the built-in flash is generally pointed directly at the subject, it will create a harsh light on the face of the subject which creates very non-flattering portraits (Fig. 12.3). For the medical photographer, the built-in lens on a camera should not be used. In fact, I have never used the built-in flash for medical photos or for my business photography. It is very easy to obtain an inexpensive external flash unit that has many more capabilities and can provide higher quality, consistent results.

I still carry an advanced compact camera for occasions when I desire high-quality photographs but do not wish to carry a large camera (Fig. 12.4). Nonetheless, the compact camera and smart phone have several important limitations, including focal length, lack of flexibility with regard to lenses, sensor size, inability to manually control settings, inability to manually control focus with precision, and resolution (in some cases). For the medical professional, the most important disadvantages are the lack of ability to manually control settings, lack of precise manual focus control, and focal length. In my mind, since portability is not of great importance when it comes to medical photography, the fixed lens/compact camera is not ideal for this purpose.

Fig. 12.3 Portrait with flash pointed directly at subject, resulting in harsh, unflattering, uneven light

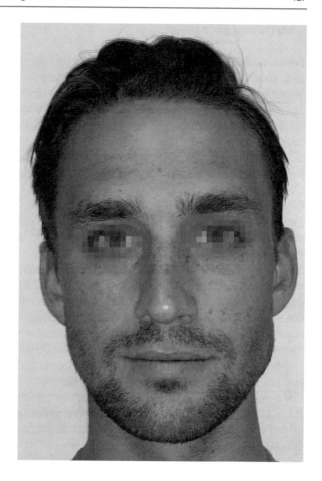

Fig. 12.4 Fixed lens/compact camera

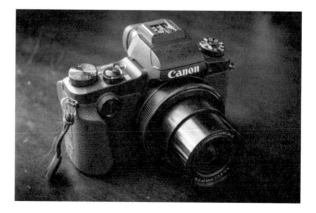

Interchangeable Lens

The interchangeable lens camera has become very popular today even among entry-level photographers. It is now a widely available product and can be obtained at a relatively low cost. It consists of a body that houses the main components of the camera itself, and a separate detachable lens. Additional accessories such as external flash units, remote controls, or wireless transmitters can often be added to these cameras, expanding the utility of the camera. Many interchangeable lens cameras also include a built-in flash, the use of which I would discourage. Interchangeable lens cameras include digital single-lens reflex and mirrorless cameras.

Digital Single-Lens Reflex vs Mirrorless

The digital single-lens-reflex (DSLR) camera is probably the most widely used type of interchangeable lens camera on the market today, and has largely replaced the 35-mm film camera. Although the mirrorless platform offers many advantages, major camera manufacturers have only recently introduced mirrorless cameras that can compete with their DSLR counterparts. Digital SLR cameras were originally developed for use with the film medium, and as the digital revolution progressed, these cameras evolved to fit the medium. Therefore, there are some major disadvantages when compared with their mirrorless counterparts. To understand these disadvantages, it is crucial to first understand how the DSLR camera functions.

When taking a picture through your smart phone or mirrorless camera, the image you see on your screen is an electronically reconstructed image based on the light that enters the lens. Light is captured on an image sensor, and this information is subsequently transferred to an electronic viewfinder (EVF) or display for viewing (Fig. 12.5). In a DSLR camera, the process is mechanically more complex. In a DSLR camera, when you look through the viewfinder (which is optical and not digital), you are seeing the light as it enters the lens, and not a digital "reconstruction" of the light data captured by an image sensor. In a DSLR camera, light enters the lens, and is reflected upwards by a reflex mirror to a pentaprism, which guides the light through the optical viewfinder. Therefore, the light entering the lens is reflected to the optical viewfinder for real-time viewing (Fig. 12.5). As such, when you look through the viewfinder on a DSLR camera, even though your eye is not lined up with the lens, you are looking through the lens because the light has been reflected by the mirror and prism.

Before the age of digital photography, image sensors were not available, and therefore viewing a digital reconstruction of an image was not possible. Cameras often required two lenses (twin lens) – one for a viewfinder, and one for a photographic objective (for capturing light on film). The advantage is that with a DSLR camera, two separate lenses (one for viewing and one for capturing the image on film/digital image sensor) are not required. However, because of this mechanism, on a DSLR camera, the photographer cannot look through the lens via the viewfinder and capture light data on the image sensor simultaneously (since the mirror is blocking the viewfinder). When the shutter is depressed on a DSLR camera, the mirror has to mechanically move out of the way of the sensor, allowing light data to pass

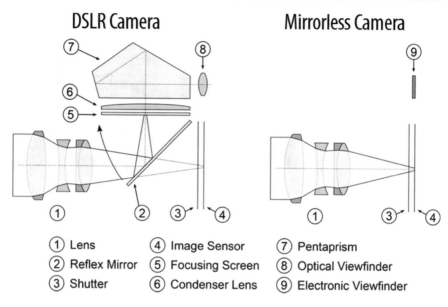

Fig. 12.5 Cross section of a mirrorless and DSLR camera. (Credit to Nasim Mansurov (https://photographylife.com/what-is-a-mirrorless-camera))

through into the sensor while momentarily blocking the image from being viewed by the user through the viewfinder. This explains why the viewfinder goes "black" when taking a photograph on a DSLR camera. This also accounts for the audible feedback when pressing the shutter, which represents the movement of the mirror and the shutter behind the mirror.

Because of the complex design of the DLSR camera, there are several key advantages and disadvantages of the camera when compared with the mirrorless camera. DSLR cameras are often bulkier because of the need to house a mirror and pentaprism (Fig. 12.5). Nonetheless, this larger size can often be beneficial when using larger lenses, or for individuals with larger hands. As discussed above, the DSLR has an optical viewfinder, permitting the photographer to view the actual light that is passing through the lens without any lag time or alteration. I personally find this helpful when taking pictures of fast-moving objects, such as wildlife. The optical viewfinder is also often better than the EVF in bright light situations. However, the EVF also has several advantages, including the ability to simulate the actual image that will be generated when the shutter is depressed, taking into account aperture, shutter speed, and ISO settings on the camera. This can be advantageous in situations when taking another shot is not possible. Additionally, the EVF has the ability to digitally display important information such as the histogram, menu settings, etc., so the photographer can make menu adjustments without looking away from the viewfinder. The DSLR camera can also be used in "Live view mode" which flips the mirror up, and permits the photographer to use the camera LCD as an electronic viewfinder. This is analogous to the electronic viewfinder on a mirrorless camera.

Fig. 12.6 Size of mirrorless (left) and DSLR (right) compared

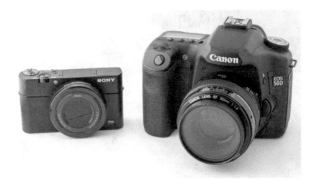

Because mirrorless camera technology is new relative to the DSLR, lens selection is often limited for mirrorless cameras. On the other hand, DSLR cameras have a wide selection of lenses. This is of particular interest to the medical photographer because lens selection is important depending on the goals of the photographer. Often times, it is useful for the medical photographer to have a macro lens, which can be difficult to obtain in some mirrorless systems at the current time. Still, some camera manufacturers have developed lens adapters, permitting DSLR lenses to be used with the newer mirrorless camera bodies. Furthermore, in the past, DSLR cameras had autofocusing systems far superior to their mirrorless counterparts, called 'phase detection' autofocus. This autofocus system can be used when the mirror in the camera is down, and is quite fast and very useful particularly when taking photographs of moving objects. The mirrorless camera uses a contrast-based autofocus system, which can be slower but in modern mirrorless cameras is more than adequate for medical photography purposes. Mirrorless cameras can also have vibration compensation technology built into the camera body, independent of the lens, which can be very useful for hand-held photography.

For my medical photos, I currently use a DSLR camera, only because this is what we had previously purchased. For my professional photos, I recently switched to the mirrorless system for several reasons, including size (Fig. 12.6) and autofocus features. For the medical professional who owns a DSLR camera, at this time there is not much to justify switching to the mirrorless system, but for the individual who does not yet have a camera, I would recommend the mirrorless camera. The compact size makes it ideal for use in clinic and the operating room, as well as for travel. The newer technology available in the mirrorless system also serves as a suitable platform for future upgrades.

Camera/Lens Attributes

Sensor Size, Focal Length, and Distortion

As discussed earlier, the electronic equivalent of film is the image sensor. Camera image sensors come in various sizes (Fig. 12.7). The image sensor of a camera

Fig. 12.7 Image
sensor sizes

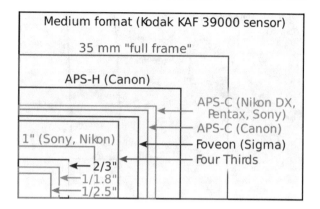

contains millions of photosites which collect light data from photons. The quality of the image that can be obtained by your camera is influenced by the type of image sensor, size of the sensor, and the number and size of the pixels on that image sensor. The image sensors on even basic, inexpensive digital cameras nowadays are more than enough to suffice for medical photography from a quality standpoint. However, image sensor size also plays a very important role in influencing field of view, which is an important consideration for lens selection and for the medical photographer. Coupled with lens focal length, image sensor size determines the angular field of view, or "35-mm equivalent focal length." This is effectively how much the camera can "see" at any given moment.

In the day of film cameras, the "sensor" (i.e., film) was of a constant size – 35 mm. Therefore, lens selection determined the angular field of view. For instance, use of a 50-mm lens on a 35-mm film camera would have a field of view calculated by the following equation:

$$a = 2\arctan\frac{d}{2f}$$

in this equation, a = angle of view, d = size of film/image sensor, f = focal length of the lens. This relationship is crucial for the medical photographer to understand because it determines what focal length lens is used for pre- and postoperative photography. Many professionals assume that focal length of the lens causes distortion. In fact, it is a common misconception that wide-angle lenses cause perspective distortion [4]. This is misleading. In reality, there are two different types of distortion that are important for the photographer – optical distortion and perspective distortion.

Optical distortion is dependent upon the optical characteristics of the particular lens being used, and can cause barrel distortion, which is a phenomenon that makes lines that are straight appear convex (Fig. 12.8). Wide-angle lenses certainly do cause optical distortion, but this is typically of such small magnitude that it has minimal consequences for the medical photographer. Thus, it is incorrect to choose a particular focal length lens assuming that it creates less distortion. The more important culprit is actually perspective distortion, which is dependent upon the

Fig. 12.8 Barrel distortion (optical)

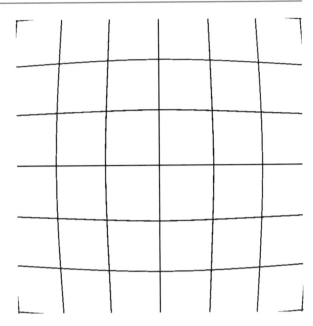

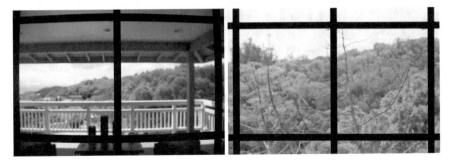

Fig. 12.9 Perspective distortion. On the left is an image taken with a 24-mm focal length at a distance of 1.5 feet from the window. The image on the right is taken with the same lens set at the same focal length at a distance of 10 feet from the window. Note the perspective distortion on the left

distance between the image sensor and the subject and independent of the optical distortion characteristics of the lens (Fig. 12.9). In Fig. 12.9, I have taken a picture of a window in my home at a distance of 1.5 feet using a 24–120-mm lens set at 24 mm and f 5.0 (left side of the figure). Notice the distortion in the lines on the window that in reality are straight. This is called *perspective distortion*. With the same lens, and the exact same settings (24 mm, f 5.0), I stepped back to a distance of 10 feet and took the picture again. I then cropped the image to demonstrate that

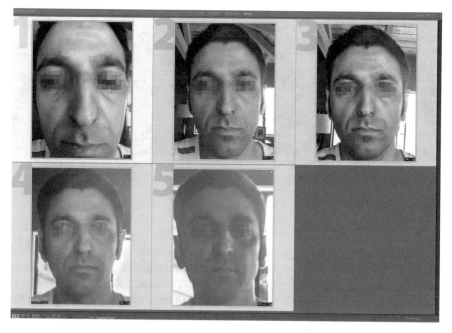

Fig. 12.10   Perspective distortion with smart phone camera

there is actually less distortion in this image because the photo was taken at a distance further away from the subject. Clearly, the distortion in the image is not because I was using a wide focal length. The distortion is a function of the distance I stood from the subject.

In Fig. 12.10, I have taken several pictures of my face using a smart phone camera to demonstrate that perspective distortion is a function of distance from the subject, and not a function of the focal length of the lens. Each of these images was taken using the same camera phone. On image 1 (top left), the camera phone is very close to my face, and in each subsequent image, I stepped back several feet. In the first image, the center of my face looks expanded, so much so that my auricles are barely visible. Compare this image with the last one in the series (labeled 5). This is evidence that focal length does not determine perspective distortion. Rather, the distance one stands from the subject is the determining factor.

Because the distance we stand from the subject is important, our angular field of view is important. Larger angular fields of view will require us to stand closer to the subject when compared with narrower angular fields of view. In the past, a 105-mm focal length lens on a standard 35-mm film camera was recommended for portrait photography (find reference). Because there are many different sensor sizes available today, we have to first know the sensor size of our camera to find the

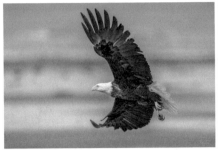

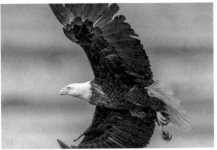

-105 mm lens → 105 mm focal
length equivalent

-105 mm lens → 157 mm focal
length equivalent

Fig. 12.11 Focal length and sensor size

appropriate lens that would provide the 35-mm film equivalent of a 105-mm focal length lens. The digital version of 35-mm film is called a "full-frame sensor." These cameras generally cost over $1000 for the body of the camera alone. On a full-frame sensor camera, a 105-mm lens will in fact result in an angular field of view similar to what you would achieve with a 105-mm lens on a 35-mm camera. Therefore, if you own a full-frame sensor camera, a 105-mm lens is an excellent choice for pre- and postoperative photography.

However, most cameras available in the market today have smaller image sensors. One of the more popular sizes of image sensors is called the "APS-C" sensor, which is substantially smaller than its full-frame counterpart. This size is also called a "cropped" sensor. Because of the smaller size of the sensor, the effective focal length of the lens is actually magnified about 1.5 times (1.6 for some manufacturers). Therefore, a 105-mm lens on a cropped sensor camera will yield a 35-mm equivalent 157-mm focal length (Fig. 12.11). This would result in a narrower angular field of view, requiring the photographer to stand further away from the subject, which can be inconvenient, particularly in the medical setting. Therefore, I generally recommend a 60-mm lens when paired with an APS-C sensor, and a 105-mm lens when paired with a full-frame sensor. I do not recommend use of a zoom lens because the adjustable focal length can introduce variability into your photography, whereas a prime (fixed focal length) lens will force the photographer to use the same focal length setting during each session, minimizing the introduction of covariates into the photographs.

Obtaining Proper Exposure

In photography, exposure is generally thought of as the amount of light that is captured by the image sensor when making a photograph. It is certainly possible to under- or overexpose a photograph (Fig. 12.12), and therefore, it is important to understand how to achieve the proper exposure. There are three major parameters

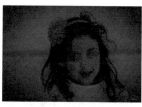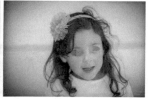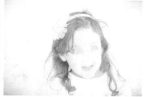

Fig. 12.12 Exposure. Under-exposed image at left, properly exposed in middle, and over-exposed at right

that can be manipulated to change the amount of light that is captured by the image sensor of your camera. These are the aperture, shutter speed, and ISO.

Aperture

The aperture setting controls how much the diaphragm of the lens opens during each exposure. The magnitude of the opening is calibrated in *f-stops*. The standard is counterintuitive, but is as follows: the lower the f-number (wide aperture), the larger the opening in the diaphragm of the lens. Conversely, the larger the f-number (narrow aperture), the smaller the opening in the lens. Consequently, a small f-number also means that more light is available to the image sensor (since the opening in the lens diaphragm is larger), while a larger f-number means that less light is available to the image sensor (since the opening in the lens diaphragm is smaller).

The aperture is also the main determinant of depth of field in a photograph. The depth of field is defined as the distance between the nearest and farthest subjects in a photograph that are in focus. This concept is of vital importance in photography, particularly when taking portraits or making images of wildlife. A low f-number will result in a shallow depth of field, which permits the photographer to isolate the object of interest from the foreground or background (Fig. 12.13 – left). This is advantageous because it directs the viewer's attention to the object of interest and prevents the image from appearing too "busy." This also provides a result that is typically pleasing to the eye. The quality of the out of focus portion of the photograph is termed "bokeh," and can also have a substantial impact on the attractiveness of an image. In some types of photography, however, it is important to keep many elements of the image in focus, regardless of their distance from one another. For instance, in a landscape, it is often helpful to keep the foreground and background in focus, which requires a high f-number (Fig. 12.13 – right). Moreover, standing closer to your subject will also create a shallower depth of field, so keep this in mind particularly when performing macro photography.

For my medical photography, I adjust my aperture based on the specific situation. For pre- and postoperative surgical photos, I generally set my aperture to be between f9 and f11. This is typically about halfway between a lens' range in terms of f-stop and is typically the "sweet spot" for the lens, providing the sharpest possible image. If more elements of the patient are required to be in focus, then the

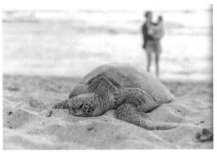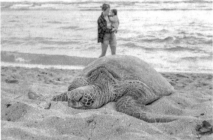

Fig. 12.13 Aperture. Image on the left shows shallow depth of field with smooth bokeh. Image on the right taken with higher f-number demonstrating wide depth of field

aperture can be stopped down (increasing the f-number) to provide more depth of field in the image as discussed earlier. Keep in mind that stopping down the aperture means that less light is available to the image sensor, so you must compensate for that loss of light by some other means.

Shutter Speed

Shutter speed is how long the image sensor is exposed to light. It is measured in seconds or fractions thereof. A lower number equates to a faster shutter speed, which means that less light is captured by the image sensor. A fast shutter speed also "freezes" a subject, thereby capturing objects in motion (Fig. 12.14 – left). On the other hand, a larger shutter speed number equates to a slower shutter speed, which can demonstrate movement (Fig. 12.14 – right). When using a slower shutter speed, a tripod is often necessary because movement of the camera would result in a blurred image, even if the subject is stationary. Many modern cameras come with vibration compensation technology built into the camera and/or the lens, which helps to reduce the effects of an unstable hand.

In general, when not using a tripod, it is beneficial to use a shutter speed at least as fast as the inverse of the focal length. For instance, if shooting with a 200-mm lens, it is best to use a shutter speed of at least 1/200th of a second. This helps to ameliorate the effects of camera shake. Vibration compensation technology can permit use of slower shutter speeds while avoiding blurring of the subject. It is important to remember that use of a fast shutter speed requires compensation by some other means to achieve proper exposure, since the light captured by the image sensor will be reduced. One option would be to open up the aperture (decrease the f-number). However, if this is not possible, using external lighting sources or changing the ISO is required. For my pre- and postoperative photographs, I typically use a shutter speed of 1/100th of a second.

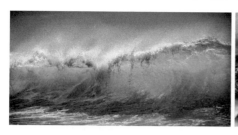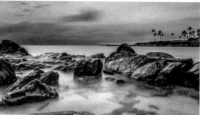

Fig. 12.14 Shutter speed. Image on the left demonstrating results of fast shutter speed. Image on the right shows effect of slower shutter speed

ISO

The camera's ISO is defined as the sensitivity of the image sensor. Each camera has a "native ISO" which is where the camera typically performs at its best. At this setting, noise in the image is typically at a minimum and dynamic range is optimized. Whereas in professional photography, this can be very important, the ISO is an area where one can be very liberal when taking photos for medical purposes. The amount of noise that is introduced into an image when not using the native ISO is quite minimal in modern cameras, and images are often of more than adequate quality.

A lower ISO means that a camera requires more light to achieve the proper exposure. Lower ISO numbers often represent the camera's native ISO. Many modern cameras have a base ISO of 100, and some have a native ISO as low as 64. Increasing the ISO means the camera's image sensor is more sensitive to light, but this occurs with a penalty. Higher ISO results in more noise in the image. Nonetheless, increasing the ISO can be beneficial in low light situations, such as nighttime. Additionally, when fast shutter speeds or narrow apertures are required (such as for fast-moving objects, or for increasing depth of field, respectively), increasing the ISO can be helpful. For medical professionals who do not have adequate external lighting, using a higher ISO can help achieve the proper exposure.

External Lighting

As previously discussed, built-in flash lighting units should be avoided as they produce flat, two-dimensional photographs. Surgical photographs should aim to produce photographs without shadows and with high depth of field. This can only be achieved with powerful external lighting sources. A set-up suitable for surgical photography is composed of two flash units positioned on either side of the camera at a 45-degree angle toward the subject. The height of the flash units should be the same as both the camera and the subject. The flash is synchronized to the camera shutter. An overhead light, referred to as a "key" light, can be positioned on the ceiling to illuminate the background. This eliminates shadowing and highlights the subject which creates a more three-dimension effect [1].

References

1. Becker DG, Tardy ME. Standardized photography in facial plastic surgery: pearls and pitfalls. Facial Plast Surg. 1999;15(02):93–9. https://doi.org/10.1055/s-2008-1064305.
2. Dey JK, Ishii LE, Nellis JC, Boahene KDO, Byrne PJ, Ishii M. Comparing patient, casual observer, and expert perception of permanent unilateral facial paralysis. JAMA Facial Plast Surg. 2017;19(6):476–83. https://doi.org/10.1001/jamafacial.2016.1630.
3. Hadlock TA, Urban LS. Toward a universal, automated facial measurement tool in facial reanimation. Arch Facial Plast Surg. 2012;14(4):277–82. https://doi.org/10.1001/archfacial.2012.111.
4. Peck JJ, Roofe SB, Kawasaki DK. Camera and lens selection for the facial plastic surgeon. Facial Plast Surg Clin North Am. 2010;18(2):223–30. https://doi.org/10.1016/j.fsc.2010.01.001.
5. Sommer DD, Mendelsohn M. Pitfalls of nonstandardized photography in facial plastic surgery patients. Plast Reconstr Surg. 2004;114(1):10–4. https://doi.org/10.1097/01.PRS.0000127791.31526.E2.

Surgical Pearls and Pitfalls

13

Lisa Ishii, Ryan M. Smith, and Matthew J. Urban

Introduction

Alopecia is a common condition with varying levels of severity that affects both men and women. Hair loss can have a negative psychosocial effect with detriments to self-esteem, social success, and perceived attractiveness. Recent evidence has proven a significant reduction in the quality of life (QOL) in patients with this condition. Health-state utility studies have demonstrated the value of treating alopecia and reveal the motivations for patients seeking treatment [1]. Surgical hair restoration is now among the most highly sought cosmetic procedures. According to the International Society for Hair Restoration Surgery (ISHRS), the number of surgical hair restoration patients increased by 109% from 2012 to 2016 and by 67% from 2014 to 2016 alone [3]. Hair restoration aims to stimulate regrowth of lost hair and unlike many medical therapies, is not limited to prevention of hair loss [2]. Tremendous advancements in hair restoration techniques have led to greatly improved outcomes since restoration was first attempted in the early 1800s [2]. Procedures in the current era include hair transplantation with follicular unit extraction (FUE) or follicular unit transplant (FUT), use of platelet-rich plasma (PRP), tissue expansion, local tissue rearrangement, and hairline lowering surgery.

As is true for any surgical procedure, and perhaps especially in cosmetic surgery, critical nuances and specifics of technique have great impact on the outcome of surgical hair restoration. Although the scalp has excellent blood supply and therefore infectious and vascular complications are rare, patient selection and preoperative education is critical. The majority of postoperative complications are preventable

L. Ishii
Johns Hopkins Hospital, Department of Otolaryngology, Lutherville, MD, USA

R. M. Smith (✉) · M. J. Urban
Facial Plastic and Reconstructive Surgery, Rush University Medical Center,
Otorhinolaryngology – Head and Neck Surgery, Chicago, IL, USA
e-mail: Ryan_m_smith@rush.edu

© Springer Nature Switzerland AG 2020
L. N. Lee (ed.), *Hair Transplant Surgery and Platelet Rich Plasma*,
https://doi.org/10.1007/978-3-030-54648-9_13

and attributed to errors in preoperative planning or surgical technique [4]. Practice management considerations including utilization of procedure room space, designating surgeon time, and incorporating technicians are rarely discussed in the literature and are of particular importance for these procedures. Patient expectations must be managed carefully, as misinformation and anecdotal reports are readily available to patients on the internet. Costly and ineffective therapies are commonly offered to patients who are highly motivated to find a solution to their hair loss [5]. In 2019, the ISHRS established the "fight the FIGHT (Fraudulent, Illicit, and Global Hair Transplants)" campaign to combat fraudulent hair restoration practices [6]. Overall, hair restoration surgery continues to gain in popularity due to its efficacy and safety. While the previous chapters have provided thorough details on hair restoration techniques, this chapter focuses on important tips, clinical pearls, and common pitfalls for surgeons performing hair restoration or hoping to incorporate this procedure into practice.

Patient Selection

While hair restoration may be beneficial to a wide range of patients, appropriate patient selection will allow the highest likelihood for success. Many authors advocate caution in patients younger than 25 years of age for multiple reasons [7]. In men with androgenetic alopecia, hair loss tends to slow after age 40 and the pattern is unpredictable while patients are in their early 20s [7]. Those who undergo hair transplantation at a younger age have greater risk for a poorly positioned hairline as they age and alopecia progresses. Future correction of this problem is challenging when prior surgery leaves an inadequate donor hair follicle supply. Younger patients also tend to seek more youthful hairlines. Treatment with topical medical therapy may temporize hair loss and delay surgical treatment until more predictable long-term outcomes can be achieved.

Hair quality is another important factor that influences the achievable result of restoration. The surgeon must account for hair shaft caliber, density, and color. Patients with hair caliber greater than 70 microns obtain a more concentrated appearance with fewer grafts. Typically, the male occiput contains 6000–10,000 donor hairs [8]. Density ranges from 80 to 100 follicular unit (FU)/cm^2, but patients with density less than 40 FU/cm^2 should be considered poor candidates. Because significant thinning may occur before clinical hair loss is evident, transplanting 25 FU/cm^2 will typically result in 50 hairs/cm^2 and give a good clinical result [7]. Patients whose hair color starkly contrasts with their skin color may require a higher density at the hairline. Individual patient factors, medical history, and expectations must be carefully considered and discussed when determining the best treatment strategy. For instance, patients who wish to wear their hair short may have difficulty camouflaging a scar from FUT. However, overharvesting by FUE may leave a "moth-eaten" appearance in the donor area [9]. A combination FUE and FUT approach may allow for greater harvesting while preserving areas for future use [9].

There are few contraindications to hair transplantation, but a detailed history and physical is necessary to proceed safely. Elective scalp surgery should be discouraged for patients with a history of bleeding disorders, hypertrophic scarring, or keloid formation. Particular populations also warrant special consideration. Non-androgenetic conditions such as lichen planopilaris or scarring alopecias, including frontal fibrosing alopecia (FFP), are clinically different from common androgenetic alopecia. These conditions may reach a "burn-out" phase at which point the condition becomes inactive and no further hair loss occurs. In this case, surgical hair restoration can safely be considered, although with caution and appropriate counseling [10].

The negative impact of hair loss on the quality of life often drives patients to seek multiple treatments until they obtain their desired outcome. It is becoming more common for patients seeking hair transplantation to have already undergone medical therapy, PRP injections, or previous procedures. The scalp should be carefully evaluated for the pattern of current hair loss, scarring, laxity, and donor follicle availability during the preoperative assessment. Counseling must include the predicted number of procedures and length of treatment necessary to reach the desired effect. FUE opens the possibility for transplanting body hair to improve the donor supply, although growth may not be as effective [9].

Lastly, it should be emphasized that grafted hair will begin to appear 3–6 months after transplantation. The process of telogen effluvium, or loss of native hair at the donor and/or recipient sites, is not uncommon. This "shock loss" is nearly always temporary, even in severe cases, and permanent loss typically signals follicles near the end of their life cycle which would have been lost anyway [4, 7]. It typically occurs in peri-incisional regions of the donor site or diffusely in the recipient bed and is likely secondary to a local inflammatory response. Recovery begins around 3 months and often coincides with when the donor follicles begin their life cycle [4]. The patient should be counseled to expect the final result with native and donor hair around 9 months post-procedure [7].

Preoperative Considerations

Multiple classification systems have been published that describe the degree and pattern of alopecia. Despite several limitations, the Norwood classification is the most widely used system worldwide. Regardless of the system used, attention to the specific anatomic regions involved must be identified in order to choose the technique that will produce the best outcome. Patients who seek treatment primarily for hair loss of the vertex should be counseled about the inherent difficulties in treating this area. Continued circumferential recession may result in a halo appearance and depletion of the donor area may leave insufficient grafts available to treat future hair loss [11]. Scalp reduction of the vertex has waned in popularity with the introduction of follicular grafting techniques, and may result in scarring with unfavorable directionality or tension [11]. Tissue expanders, previously favored to treat the vertex, are uncomfortable and may thin hair density in donor areas [11]. Temporal recession and attention to the current condition of the hairline is an important consideration, as is managing expectations of these areas after treatment.

Available Technology

Technological advancements have revolutionized the process of hair transplantation since its inception. The concept of implanting individual follicular units drastically improved the aesthetic result upon introduction in the 1990s [12]. In 2011, the Food and Drug Administration approved the first robotic technology in dermatologic surgery [12]. This was designed to improve efficiency and increase graft survival rate by decreasing the rate of follicular transection and the overall time that grafts exist ex vivo. Unlike other robotic surgical technologies, these have the capacity to work independent of an operator. These systems use fiducials to guide the isolation of individual follicular units and extract them with a low rate of transection. This rate has been demonstrated to equal that of a trained surgical team performing the same operation [13]. Lasers are also adapted for use in hair transplantation and their use continues to evolve.

Procedural Pearls and Pitfalls

Graft Harvest

Selecting the ideal harvest site is the critical first step in surgical hair restoration. Typically, hair-bearing scalp located below the occiput and extending laterally to the edge of the helix is chosen as the donor site [8]. Placement of the donor site too high may cause harvest of follicles susceptible to the androgenetic process resulting in poor outcomes. Placement too low risks a visible or elongated scar if FUT techniques are used [4].

Ideal positioning of the patient during harvest will ensure their comfort and improve the ease of the procedure. An upright or prone position with a cushioned C-shaped headrest can work well. Prone positioning has the advantage of maximal patient comfort while also decreasing the likelihood of a fall in the event of a vasovagal episode. Patient satisfaction with the overall procedure may be improved if entertainment options such as reading materials, music, or television are offered. Certain positions preclude this but ultimately whichever position enables the best quality harvest should be used.

Careful preparation of the harvest site is essential. Proper anesthesia of the scalp provides patient comfort, increases technical ease, reduces total procedure time, and ensures harvest of quality grafts. Local anesthesia is of increased importance for hair transplantation as the scalp is highly sensitive and vascular. Transplantation procedures are typically lengthy and fine attention to detail is required. Surgical techniques become increasingly difficult in a bloody field or with an uncomfortable patient. Use of sedation and general anesthesia can be avoided with thorough injections of local anesthesia, which can be injected at intervals while monitoring total dose. The use of regional nerve blocks should be considered as they allow a lower total dose of local and provide excellent pain control. The supraorbital and supratrochlear nerves are the most commonly targeted. Distracting bleeding due to the rich vascularity of the scalp can be lessened by using local with vasoconstricting components. One formulation described by Epstein et al. [9] contains 50 mL of saline, 10 mL of 0.5% bupivacaine, 0.5 mL of 1:1000 epinephrine, and 0.4 mL of triamcinolone acetate.

After the site is prepared, harvest can proceed. Several technical considerations can improve the quality of the result. The directionality of hair follicles must be inspected and appreciated in order to avoid transection during harvest. For strip excision in FUT, the surgeon should take care to incise parallel to follicles to avoid transection. Undermining should be limited to the amount necessary to allow a tension-free wound closure as excessive undermining may cause scar fibrosis and reduced scalp laxity which can limit subsequent procedures [7].

The use of trichophytic closure of the strip excision site has been well supported in the literature and in practice. Trichophytic closure allows for donor scar camouflage and was first described by Marzola [14]. Briefly, one side of the incision is sharply trimmed in a beveled manner approximately 1–2 mm from the skin edge with care to avoid transection of adjacent hair follicle bulbs. Limited undermining is performed to reduce tension and the skin edges are meticulously approximated with sutures. This technique allows the non-beveled skin edge to overlap the closure. This preserves hair-bearing scalp adjacent to the incision and redirects the growth of hair follicles in the beveled skin towards and through the scar. This helps to prevent a hairless gap and noticeable scar.

Graft harvest in FUE restoration has a higher rate of follicular transection compared to FUT, likely because strip harvest in FUT provides a single, larger segment of scalp containing relatively undisturbed follicles. FUE is commonly chosen to avoid a potentially unsightly donor scar, and therefore separate, smaller grafts are harvested. This increases the potential for transection around the periphery of each graft. To minimize transection during FUE, varying amounts of pressure should be applied by the punch to the skin. Initially, light pressure should be used to puncture the epidermis but limit sharp transection of surrounding hair follicles. Increased pressure can be applied when the leading edge of the punch is below the level of the hair follicles in the deep dermis or subcutaneous layer. Recent advancements in robotic technology such as oscillating drill mechanisms that can be controlled with foot pedals may decrease surrounding tissue injury and lower transection rates in FUE.

Graft Preparation

Regardless of the harvest method, preparation of individual follicular grafts for re-implantation must be done with care. This is a tedious and time-consuming process that introduces the risk of non-viability after placement in the recipient location.

Several factors during graft preparation may damage the follicles or lead to loss after implantation including thermal damage, ischemia, metabolic deficiencies, or reperfusion injury. Several bioenhancement mediums are available and designed to limit damage from these factors by providing an ionically balanced environment and hypothermic conditions for grafts during preparation. Metabolic factors, pH control, and antioxidants are often components of these mediums and some include growth factors meant to nurture recently implanted grafts during the time it takes for revascularization to occur. Ultimately, there is no substitute for careful planning and atraumatic technique.

A well-planned and efficiently performed procedure may limit the time spent out of the body and improve outcomes. Practice management considerations will be discussed later in this chapter and are particularly applicable to graft preparation and the quality and viability of grafts ready for re-implantation.

Graft Implantation

Graft placement is an exacting science that requires forethought and precise execution. Recipient incisions must be placed in optimal locations and in a manner that will best accommodate the implanted graft. Early surgical restoration procedures used the sagittal technique of creating incisions parallel to the direction of hair growth. However, the lateral slit technique, in which recipient incisions are placed at an angle of approximately 30–45 degrees, more closely replicates the natural direction of hair growth. This may also allow greater overall coverage of the treated area as the exit angle and direction of each graft can be controlled by the recipient incision. Development of surgical blades that approximate the size of a single follicular unit allow precise incisions of optimal depth and width which cause less trauma to the recipient scalp tissues and implanted follicles.

Blunt or transecting trauma to follicular grafts can occur while grasping them for insertion or while advancing the grafts into the recipient incision. Jeweler's forceps are often used during implantation and it is critical to avoid follicular damage by grasping each follicle with gentle pressure. Grasping too tightly can cause transection or damage leading to follicle death after implantation. Ideally, grafts are placed within incisions in a single attempt, as multiple attempts are more likely to cause injury. The availability of implantation instruments with the multifunctionality to create the recipient incision, deliver the follicle, and advance it to the appropriate depth may reduce the need for multiple attempts and decrease trauma.

Postoperative Considerations

An overnight dressing is applied and the patient is given a short course of oral steroids to reduce surgical site edema. Pain is usually very mild and our practice typically dispenses five acetaminophen-codeine tablets. Patients are instructed to apply topical emollients such as petrolatum or mineral oil-based ointments for 7 days to prevent dehydration of grafts within the recipient environment. It is important to remember that grafts are not fully vascularized until several days after implantation and survive by the process of inosculation prior to this. Mild crusting at the recipient sites is expected and can be gently cleansed but significant crusting if emollients are not used can impede viability. Showering is permitted on the first postoperative day and patients should allow water to gently rinse over their scalp without applying pressure or soaking the area. Patients are counseled not to expect results for 8–12 months. A thorough preoperative discussion with clear communication and management of expectations can reduce postoperative anxiety about the outcome. Specifically, the phenomenon of telogen effluvium should be explained to the patient as a temporary condition that usually occurs around 3 months postoperatively and may last up to 6 months in duration. Wound healing issues and noticeable scarring can occur even if trichophytic closure is performed. Therefore, close follow-up and early intervention with topical therapies and corticosteroid treatments should be considered to manage the appearance of the scar if issues arise. Standard clinical photography should be utilized throughout the restoration process to document the findings at each visit. Additionally, detailed records of the technique utilized, number of follicular units implanted, adjuvant therapies prescribed, and other relevant details should be documented. This information not only informs the long-term treatment of an individual patient, but also drives the development of the restoration surgeon's skill and outcomes over the course of their career.

Practice Management

Particular practice management considerations are important when incorporating hair restoration surgery into practice. Surgical restoration procedures are typically lengthy and at least initially may need to be performed with limited support. A successful practice must optimize efficiency without compromising safety or quality. Procedural timing during the surgeon's daily schedule should be carefully planned. Critical portions should be completed safely and swiftly while the entirety of the procedure is managed to allow for additional clinical, administrative, or academic productivity during down time. Many, but not all, practices employ technicians for the microscopic follicular unit grafting portions of the procedure. The ISHRS reports that among 100 practices surveyed, the average number of technicians employed is 5 with a range from 0 to 25 [2]. It is our opinion that in order to ensure patient safety, the surgeon should directly oversee mapping of the recipient area, designating and harvesting the donor tissue, and closing the harvest sites. In many cases, expert technicians with vast experience handling and preparing follicular grafts not only improve efficiency but also contribute to excellent outcomes.

References

1. Abt NB, Quatela O, Heiser A, Jowett N, Tessler O, Lee LN. Association of hair loss with health utility measurements before and after hair transplant surgery in men and women. JAMA Facial Plast Surg. 2018;20(6):495. https://doi.org/10.1001/JAMAFACIAL.2018.1052.
2. Stoneburner J, Shauly O, Carey J, Patel KM, Stevens WG, Gould DJ. Contemporary management of alopecia: a systematic review and meta-analysis for surgeons. Aesthet Plast Surg. 2020;44(1):97–113. https://doi.org/10.1007/s00266-019-01529-9.
3. International Society of Hair Restoration Surgery: 2017 Practice Census Results. https://ishrs.org/wp-content/uploads/2017/12/report_2017_ishrs_practice_census-08-21-17.pdf. Published 2017. Accessed 29 Apr 2020.
4. Nadimi S. Complications with hair transplantation. Facial Plast Surg Clin North Am. 2020;28(2):225–35. https://doi.org/10.1016/j.fsc.2020.01.003.
5. Ishii LE, Lee LN. Hair transplantation: advances in diagnostics, artistry, and surgical techniques. Facial Plast Surg Clin North Am. 2020;28(2):xi–xii. https://doi.org/10.1016/j.fsc.2020.02.001.
6. ISHRS launches fight the FIGHT public awareness campaign to combat fraudulent hair restoration practices worldwide – ISHRS. https://ishrs.org/2019/11/01/ishrs-launches-fight-the-fight-public-awareness-campaign/. Published 2019. Accessed 29 Apr 2020.
7. Sand JP. Follicular unit transplantation. Facial Plast Surg Clin North Am. 2020;28(2):161–7. https://doi.org/10.1016/j.fsc.2020.01.005.
8. Rawnsley JD. Hair restoration. Facial Plast Surg Clin North Am. 2008;16(3):289–97. https://doi.org/10.1016/j.fsc.2008.04.002.
9. Epstein GK, Epstein J, Nikolic J. Follicular unit excision: current practice and future developments. Facial Plast Surg Clin North Am. 2020;28(2):169–76. https://doi.org/10.1016/j.fsc.2020.01.006.
10. Lee JA, Levy DA, Patel KG, Brennan E, Oyer SL. Hair transplantation in frontal fibrosing alopecia and lichen planopilaris: a systematic review. Laryngoscope. 2020:1–8. https://doi.org/10.1002/lary.28551.
11. Devroye J. Management of the crown. Facial Plast Surg Clin North Am. 2013;21(3):397–406. https://doi.org/10.1016/j.fsc.2013.06.005.
12. Avram MR, Watkins S. Robotic hair transplantation. Facial Plast Surg Clin North Am. 2020;28(2):189–96. https://doi.org/10.1016/j.fsc.2020.01.011.
13. Shin JW, Kwon SH, Kim SA, et al. Characteristics of robotically harvested hair follicles in Koreans. J Am Acad Dermatol. 2015;72(1):146–50. https://doi.org/10.1016/j.jaad.2014.07.058.
14. Marzola M. Trichophytic closure of the donor area. Hair Transplant Forum Int. 2005;15:113.

Index

© Springer Nature Switzerland AG 2020
L. N. Lee (ed.), *Hair Transplant Surgery and Platelet Rich Plasma*,
https://doi.org/10.1007/978-3-030-54648-9

Printed in the United States
by Baker & Taylor Publisher Services